THE
PHYSICIAN
ASSISTANT
STUDENT'S
GUIDE
to the Clinical Year

OB/GYN

Elyse Watkins, DHSc, PA-C, DFAAPA, is an associate professor for the Doctor of Medical Science (DMSc) program at the University of Lynchburg's School of PA Medicine, where she teaches women's health, global health, and evidence-based medicine. She is also a visiting lecturer at Florida State University, where she teaches the women's health module to physician assistant (PA) students. She works clinically per diem for Wake Forest Baptist Community Physicians in Winston-Salem, North Carolina. Dr. Watkins has worked in PA education since 2012, serving in both the clinical and didactic phases of PA curricula. She speaks at state, regional, and national continuing medical education (CME) conferences on women's health topics, has published several articles in *Journal of the American Academy of Physician Assistants* (*JAAPA*), and has written two books and one chapter in peer-reviewed clinical books. She is active in local, state, and national PA organizations. She has also worked with several state and regional organizations to advocate for greater utilization of PAs in obstetrics and gynecology practices. She graduated from the George Washington University's PA program in 1993. She also has a BA in anthropology and sociology and an MSc in healthcare management. She earned her DHSc with a concentration in global health from Nova Southeastern University in 2016. She was a National Health Service Corps Scholarship recipient and fulfilled her commitment to practice in a Central California migrant clinic in 1995. The majority of her clinical career has been spent working in obstetrics and gynecology in the Central Valley of California, and she has completed medical missions to Nicaragua, Guatemala, and Tanzania.

Maureen Knechtel, MPAS, PA-C (Series Editor), received a bachelor's degree in health science and a master's degree in physician assistant (PA) studies from Duquesne University in Pittsburgh, Pennsylvania. She is the author of the textbook *EKGs for the Nurse Practitioner and Physician Assistant*, first and second editions. Ms. Knechtel is a fellow member of the Physician Assistant Education Association, the American Academy of Physician Assistants, and the Tennessee Academy of Physician Assistants. She is the academic coordinator and an assistant professor for the Milligan College Physician Assistant Program in Johnson City, Tennessee, and practices as a cardiology PA with the Ballad Health Cardiovascular Associates Heart Institute. Ms. Knechtel has been a guest lecturer nationally and locally on topics including EKG interpretation, chronic angina, ischemic and hemorrhagic stroke, hypertension, and mixed hyperlipidemia.

THE PHYSICIAN ASSISTANT STUDENT'S GUIDE
to the Clinical Year

OB/GYN

Elyse Watkins, DHSc, PA-C, DFAAPA

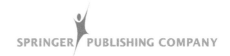

SPRINGER PUBLISHING COMPANY

Copyright © 2020 Springer Publishing Company, LLC

Springer Publishing Company, LLC
11 West 42nd Street
New York, NY 10036
www.springerpub.com
http://connect.springerpub.com/home

Acquisitions Editor: Suzanne Toppy
Compositor: diacriTech

ISBN: 978-0-8261-9526-5
ebook ISBN: 978-0-8261-9536-4
DOI: 10.1891/9780826195364

21 22 23 / 10 9 8 7

The author and the publisher of this Work have made every effort to use sources believed to be reliable to provide information that is accurate and compatible with the standards generally accepted at the time of publication. Because medical science is continually advancing, our knowledge base continues to expand. Therefore, as new information becomes available, changes in procedures become necessary. We recommend that the reader always consult current research and specific institutional policies before performing any clinical procedure or delivering any medication. The author and publisher shall not be liable for any special, consequential, or exemplary damages resulting, in whole or in part, from the readers' use of, or reliance on, the information contained in this book. The publisher has no responsibility for the persistence or accuracy of URLs for external or third-party Internet websites referred to in this publication and does not guarantee that any content on such websites is, or will remain, accurate or appropriate.

CIP data is on file at the Library of Congress.
Library of Congress Control Number: 2019911084

Contact us to receive discount rates on bulk purchases.
We can also customize our books to meet your needs.
For more information please contact: sales@springerpub.com

Publisher's Note: New and used products purchased from third-party sellers are not guaranteed for quality, authenticity, or access to any included digital components.

Printed in the United States of America.

Contents

e-Chapter 10. Case Studies in OB/GYN
http://connect.springerpub.com/content/book/978-0-8261-9536
-4/chapter/ch10

e-Chapter 11. Review Questions in OB/GYN
http://connect.springerpub.com/content/book/978-0-8261-9536
-4/chapter/ch11

Peer Reviewer

Alison McLellan, MMS, PA-C, Associate Professor, School of Physician Assistant Studies, College of Health Professions, Pacific University, Forest Grove, Oregon. *Alison McLellan is an item writer for the Physician Assistant Education Association (PAEA) PACKRAT Exam Development Board and did not write or review any practice questions for this book.*

Foreword

The Physician Assistant Student's Guide to the Clinical Year: OB/GYN is a must-read for the student who will be learning how to provide healthcare to women of all ages. This book presents all the clinically relevant, evidence-based, and best practice guidelines in a concise, understandable, and well-organized fashion. I have been blessed to have worked with the author in the clinical setting and witnessed the excellence, passion, and consistency that she possesses. Dr. Watkins's collective knowledge and substantial experience are reflected in this invaluable resource, which walks you through the most common problems you will encounter when taking care of women. These issues are presented in a concise format that describes the cause, clinical presentation, diagnosis, and management in a manner that is easy to remember. This book enables you to deliver excellent care on your way to becoming an experienced clinician.

A first of its kind, this book is a much-needed resource for physician assistant students about to embark on their clinical rotation in OB/GYN. Incorporating the tools in this book into your daily practice will provide a solid resource and help form a solid foundation for the new clinician, resulting in excellent care to women.

CARY SHAKESPEARE, MD

Preface

For a physician assistant student, the clinical year marks a time of great excitement and anticipation. It is a time to hone the skills you have learned in your didactic training and work toward becoming a competent and confident healthcare provider. After many intense semesters in the classroom, you will have the privilege of participating in the practice of medicine. Each rotation will reinforce, refine, and enhance your knowledge and skills through exposure and repetition. When you look back on this time, you will likely relish the opportunities, experiences, and people involved along the way. You may find an affinity for a medical specialty you did not realize you enjoyed. You will meet lifelong professional mentors and friends. You may even be hired for your first job.

Although excitement is the overlying theme, some amount of uncertainty is bound to be present as you progress from rotation to rotation, moving through the various medical specialties. You have gained a vast knowledge base during your didactic training, but you may be unsure of how to utilize it in a fast-paced clinical environment. As a clinical year physician assistant student, you are not expected to know everything, but you are expected to seek out resources that can complement what you will learn through hands-on experience. Through an organized and predictable approach, this book series serves as a guide and companion to help you feel prepared for what you will encounter during the clinical year.

Each book was written by physician assistant educators, clinicians, and preceptors who are experts in their respective fields. Their knowledge from years of experience is laid out in the pages before you. Each book will answer questions such as "What does my preceptor want me to know?" "What should I be familiar with prior to this rotation?" and "What can I expect to encounter during this rotation?" This is followed by a guided approach to the clinical decision-making process for common presenting complaints, detailed explanations of common disease entities, and specialty-specific patient education.

Chapters are organized in a way that will allow you to quickly access vital information that can help you recognize, diagnose, and treat commonly seen conditions. You can easily review suggested labs and diagnostic imaging for a suspected diagnosis, find a step-by-step guide to frequently performed procedures, and review urgent management of conditions specific to each rotation. Electronic resources are available for each book. These include case studies with explanations to evaluate your clinical reasoning process, and review questions to assist in self-evaluation and preparation for your end-of-rotation examinations as well as the Physician Assistant National Certifying Exam.

As a future physician assistant, you have already committed to being a lifelong learner of medicine. It is my hope that this book series will outline expectations, enhance your medical knowledge base, and provide you with the confidence you need to be successful in your clinical year.

MAUREEN KNECHTEL, **MPAS, PA-C**
Series Editor
The Physician Assistant Student's Guide to the Clinical Year

Acknowledgments

To my children, Ryan, Jackson, and Robert, thank you for giving me the space and time to write this book. I love you more than you can imagine.

To my physicians, Armi Walker and Cary Shakespeare, thank you for believing in me and giving me the freedom to walk this journey.

To my patients who have allowed me to help care for them during some of the most intimate, heartbreaking, and soul-filling events of their lives, thank you for trusting me. I am humbled beyond words.

To my former PA students, thank you for challenging me and helping me become a better teacher.

Finally, to Maureen Knechtel, thank you for presenting the idea for this series to Springer Publishing Company, staying committed to its success, and allowing me to write about what I love.

ELYSE WATKINS

Introduction

The Approach to the Patient in Obstetrics and Gynecology

WHAT TO EXPECT

Welcome to your women's health rotation. Some of you will have rotations in public health departments, outpatient clinics, or a combination of outpatient and inpatient experiences. Regardless of where you are placed, this book provides you with invaluable tips, pearls, and "must-knows."

The most important piece of advice that can be offered to you initially is to have a positive attitude. Many former students went into their OB/GYN rotation with dread and trepidation. Remember that you will likely encounter patients with women's health-related issues while on primary care rotations, on emergency medicine rotations, and in urgent care settings, so it is not limited to just the OB/GYN setting. Some students have expressed frustration because they knew they wanted to practice orthopedics or cardiovascular surgery, for example, and did not want to have to do anything related to women's health. Success on all rotations requires a positive attitude and a willingness to learn.

It is important to reach out to your contact person at the site to ask about dress code expectations. For example, should you wear your own scrubs to clinic? If you are going to be able to first assist and/or assist with vaginal deliveries, you will be able to utilize the hospital scrubs that will be available to you. Please keep in mind that a lot of your time will be spent sitting on a stool during clinic. As such, women, please do not wear short skirts, and on the contrary, extra-long skirts can get caught in the wheels of the stool. You also may want to rethink wearing your best outfits to clinic because there is a chance you will have urine, blood, and even feces spill on you.

If you are going to have hospital experiences, think about bringing a pair of medical clogs or clean sneakers that you can change into when you go from clinic to hospital. Never wear open-toe shoes to clinic or the hospital.

Long fingernails, particularly if painted, are not recommended. Remember that you will be wearing gloves during exams and in the operating room, so consider not wearing rings or other jewelry that you will have to remove. Rings, and even plain bands, can harbor harmful bacteria that can adversely affect your patients. If you have not yet been involved in a surgical rotation, remember that you will need to wear hats during deliveries and in the operating room. As such, consider wearing your hair pulled back and be prepared to have "hat head" after longer cases.

Some students are sensitive to the smells inherent in OB/GYN. Retained tampons, for example, can be so malodorous that the room may need to be closed until the garbage can be taken out. While performing pelvic exams, you will be sitting right next to the patient's feet. Some patients have particularly malodorous feet. One way to mitigate the reaction you may have to some of these odors is to have a small bottle of an essential oil that you find pleasant smelling. Place a dab of oil under your nostrils. The essential oil can also be used during deliveries as some students have an aversion to the smell of placenta and blood in general.

Bring your stethoscope with you. Many OB/GYN offices may only have one or two spare stethoscopes lying around, and if so, they are likely to be a lower grade model, not top-of-the-line cardiology stethoscopes. Patients who come to the OB/GYN office still need to have their hearts and lungs checked, when appropriate. You may want to bring your reflex hammer and ophthalmoscope as well (more on that later). As in any healthcare facility, please make sure you clean your instruments on a regular basis. Helping reduce healthcare-associated infections by cleaning your instruments (and washing your hands) is everyone's responsibility.

If you are afforded the opportunity to first or second assist and/or attend deliveries, make sure you do not wear worn scrubs out of the hospital. In addition, please make sure your lab coat is clean on the first day of your rotation. You should wash it at least weekly.

It is a good idea to ask a few nurses on the floor if you can spend time with them. The labor and delivery nurses are usually very good about reinforcing concepts regarding progression through labor, how to read the tocometer, and dealing with uncomplicated delivery in general. It may be well worth your time to spend a night shift with the nurses.

CLINICAL PEARL: Always have a gestation wheel in your lab coat pocket and learn how to use it.

WHAT YOUR PRECEPTOR WANTS YOU TO KNOW

THE MENSTRUAL CYCLE

There are several components of the normal menstrual cycle. See Box I.1 and Box I.2 for descriptions of the menstrual cycle. The endometrium and the ovaries go through changes throughout the cycle. The proliferative endometrium occurs after the previous cycle's sloughing and during the ovarian follicular phase. Ovulation occurs after the luteinizing hormone (LH) surge during the midcycle, ushering in the luteal phase of the ovarian cycle. Once ovulation occurs, the endometrium becomes highly vascularized. This change is due to the influence of estrogen and progesterone. Remember that progesterone is secreted by the corpus luteum. As the endometrium becomes more tortuous, it secretes a clear fluid, hence its name, secretory phase. If pregnancy does not occur, the corpus luteum begins regression. This process results in endometrial hormonal withdrawal, and menstruation ensues. The average length of the menstrual cycle is 3 to 5 days, and the average amount of blood loss equals about 30 mL. Keep in mind that some women will bleed much less and others will bleed more.

> **CLINICAL PEARL:** Some patients will be convinced that they are hemorrhaging with each cycle. The best way to evaluate abnormal blood loss in the nonemergent setting is with a hemoglobin and hematocrit.

Box I.1 Characteristics of Each Menstrual Phase

- Early follicular: FSH increases, LH gradually increases, and E2 and progesterone (P) are low.
- Late follicular: Follicle begins to mature, FSH decreases, inhibin increases, and estradiol increases.
- Ovulatory: Ovum release occurs, E2 levels peak, P increases, and LH surge occurs.
- Luteal: Dominant follicle that releases ovum becomes corpus luteum; E2, P, and inhibin increase; and LH and FSH decrease.

E2, estradiol; FSH, follicle-stimulating hormone; LH, luteinizing hormone.

The endometrium undergoes transitions during the menstrual cycle as well. Endometrial biopsies and Papanicolaou (Pap) testing that contains endometrial tissue will report on which phase is present at the time of sampling.

Box I.2 Characteristics of Each Endometrial Phase

- *Menstrual phase*: Day 1 to the first 4 or 5 days of bleeding
- *Proliferative phase*: Endometrial proliferation secondary to estradiol stimulation
- *Secretory phase*: Corpus luteum secretes progesterone, which stimulates endometrial glandular cells

---

If fertilization and pregnancy do not occur by about day 23, the corpus luteum undergoes regression, thus decreasing the amount of progesterone and estradiol, resulting in menstruation (Figure I.1).

The term *dysfunctional uterine bleeding* has fallen out of favor. The American College of Obstetricians and Gynecologists recommends using the term *abnormal uterine bleeding* (AUB) instead. Remember, AUB is a symptom that requires an etiology. Irregular bleeding can be called *AUB* when the bleeding is not caused from hematologic disorders, pharmacologic interventions, trauma,

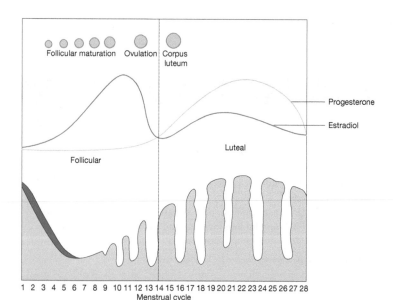

FIGURE I.1 The menstrual cycle: Schematic of the ovary depicting the developing follicle and oocyte in the ovarian cortex.

malignancy, systemic disease, and pregnancy. AUB is classified using the PALM-COEIN system. PALM is the acronym for the structural causes of AUB, which stands for **p**olyp, **a**denomyosis, **l**eiomyoma, and **m**alignancy and hyperplasia. COEIN is the acronym for the nonstructural causes of AUB, which stands for **c**oagulopathy, **o**vulatory dysfunction, **e**ndometrial, **i**atrogenic, and **n**ot otherwise classified. See Chapter 2, Common Disease Entities in Gynecology.

> **CLINICAL PEARL:** Heavy bleeding in an adolescent should prompt a von Willebrand workup, and any bleeding in a postmenopausal patient requires a workup for endometrial hyperplasia and cancer.

GYNECOLOGIC ANATOMY

Inspection and palpation of the breasts must include the nipples, areola, skin, breast tissue, and lymph nodes (Figure I.2). Always check for asymmetry, skin changes, and obvious deformities. Document the presence of scars. Remember that the axillary lymph nodes must be palpated bilaterally, as should the infra- and supraclavicular lymph nodes.

The external genitalia consist of bilateral vulva, the urethra, the clitoris, Skene's glands, Bartholin glands, the introitus, and the perineum (Figures I.3 and I.4).

> **CLINICAL PEARL:** No two women's external genitalia is the same.

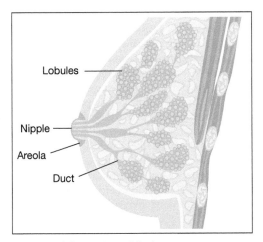

Lobules

Nipple

Areola

Duct

FIGURE I.2 Anatomical illustration of the breast.

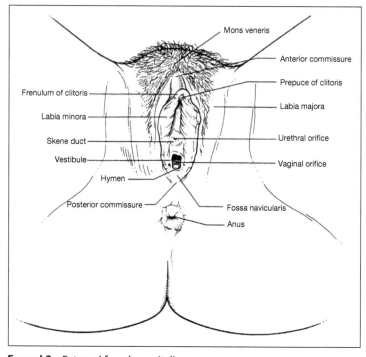

FIGURE I.3 External female genitalia.
Source: From Carcio HA, Secor RM. *Advanced Health Assessment of Women: Clinical Skills and Procedures.* 4th ed. New York, NY: Springer Publishing Company; 2019:4.

The uterus is supported by four sets of ligaments (Figure I.5). The round ligaments help to maintain the position of the uterus in the pelvis but do not affect uterine prolapse. During pregnancy, it is not uncommon for women to have sharp pelvic pain either on both sides or on one side of the pelvis. *Round ligament pain is the leading cause of nonpathologic pelvic pain during pregnancy.* The uterosacral ligaments provide sympathetic and parasympathetic innervation to the uterus. The cardinal ligaments help prevent uterine prolapse. The pubocervical ligaments attach the cervix to the pubic symphysis. The broad ligament is attached to the uterus, ovaries, and fallopian tubes. Within the broad ligament are three other ligaments: the ovarian ligament, the round ligament, and the infundibulopelvic ligament.

Vasculature of the external genitalia primarily occurs from the branches of the pudendal artery. The innervation of the external genitalia is by the pudendal nerve. The vagina is, on average, 8 cm deep. Menopause and hysterectomy can shorten the vaginal canal (Figures I.6 and I.7).

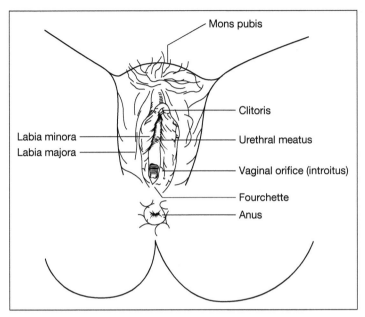

FIGURE I.4   Anatomy of the vulva.

Source: From Carcio HA, Secor RM. *Advanced Health Assessment of Women: Clinical Skills and Procedures.* 4th ed. New York, NY: Springer Publishing Company; 2019:84.

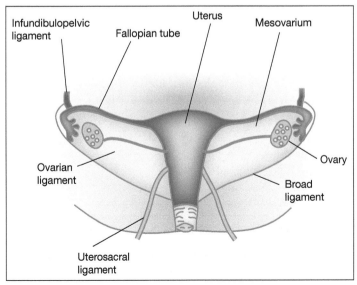

FIGURE I.5   The pelvic ligaments in the postnatal female.

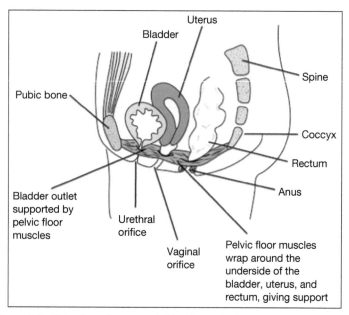

FIGURE I.6 Side view of a woman's bladder and related structures.

Note how the urethral and vaginal orifices and rectum pass through the strap of the pelvic muscles.

Source: From Carcio HA, Secor RM. *Advanced Health Assessment of Women: Clinical Skills and Procedures.* 4th ed. New York, NY: Springer Publishing Company; 2019:66.

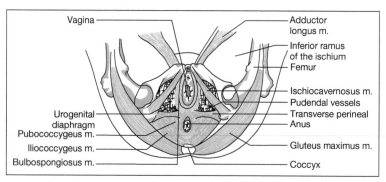

FIGURE I.7 Anatomy and musculature of the pelvic floor.

m., muscle.

Source: From Secor RM, Fantasia HC. *Fast Facts about the Gynecologic Exam.* 2nd ed. New York, NY: Springer Publishing Company; 2018:35.

Some women may have undergone a cultural procedure called *female genital cutting* or *mutilation* while they were young and unable to provide informed consent. This practice is endemic to some areas of Africa, Indonesia, and the Middle East. The practice is illegal in the United States (Figure I.8).

The vaginal walls have folds, called *rugae*. Rugae are responsive to estrogen, so when a woman is oopherectomized or menopausal, the rugae decrease, and the vagina becomes less elastic and appears pale. This finding is called *atrophic vaginitis*. The cervix is a part of the uterus. The average length of the cervix is 3 cm. The opening of the cervix is called the *os*. The os has an internal and external component. You must understand this because when you are performing cervical checks for dilation and effacement on pregnant patients, you may need to differentiate between the internal and external os. The squamocolumnar junction depends upon a patient's hormonal status. Premenarchal, the ectocervix is composed of squamous cells. Once menstruation occurs, under the influence of estrogen, the external os will open slightly, exposing

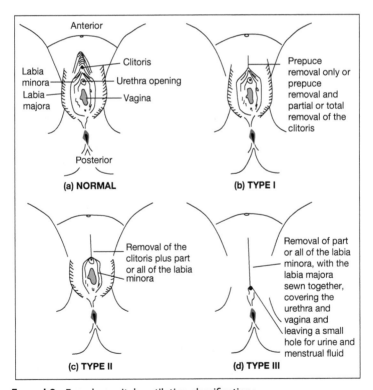

Figure I.8 Female genital mutilation classifications.

Source: From Secor RM, Fantasia HC. *Fast Facts About the Gynecologic Exam.* 2nd ed. New York, NY: Springer Publishing Company; 2018:123.

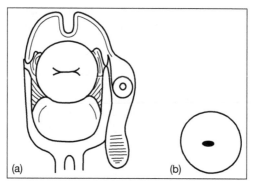

Figure I.9 Inspecting the cervix. (a) Multiparous cervix. (b) Nulliparous cervix.

Source: From Secor RM, Fantasia HC. *Fast Facts about the Gynecologic Exam.* 2nd ed. New York, NY: Springer Publishing Company; 2018:46.

columnar cells. This is referred to as *ectropion*. The area where columnar cells replace squamous cells is referred to as the *transformation zone*. Over the course of the reproductive life span, squamous cells will replace the columnar cells (Figure I.9).

The ovaries average 3 cm × 2 cm × 2 cm. Blood supply is via the long ovarian arteries inferior to the renal arteries and the uterine artery. Venous drainage of the left ovary is through the left renal vein, and venous drainage from the right ovary is through the inferior vena cava.

The abdominal ureters lie posteriorly to the broad ligament. During intra-abdominal and pelvic surgeries, it is important to identify the ureters so they are not nicked.

There are several layers of the lower abdominal wall that you must be able to identify when you are first or second assisting in surgery. The layers, in order, are as follows:

- Skin
- Subcutaneous fat
- Superficial fascia
- Deep fascia
- Anterior rectus sheath (This is a strong white sheet of fibrous tissue that connects the lateral abdominal wall muscles. It meets in the midline of the inner abdomen to create the linea alba.)

If you have the opportunity to first assist in surgery, you will encounter various abdominal wall incisions.

- Pfannenstiel: This is the most common incision. It is a horizontal curved incision about 2 cm above the symphysis pubis. This incision avoids the rectus abdominus incision, so hernias rarely develop.

- Lower midline (vertical): Occurs about 2 cm above the symphysis pubis. It is a vertical incision to below the umbilicus.
- Transverse (Maylard, Bardenheuer): This incision type is primarily used for extensive pelvic surgeries such as in patients with gynecologic malignancy.

> **CLINICAL PEARL:** It is a good idea to review the pelvic anatomy and abdominal wall layers prior to going to the operating room.

OB/GYN physicians follow the guidelines of the American College of Obstetricians and Gynecologists (ACOG) regarding common OB/GYN conditions. You can access ACOG's Practice Bulletins via your school's medical library. Be prepared to discuss a practice guideline if you have been asked to read about a topic.

When presenting a patient to your preceptor, remember that OB/GYNs are busy people and it is possible that they have been up all night with laboring patients, performing emergency cesarean surgeries, and consulting in the ED. Be clear, concise, and as quick as you can. As a general rule, begin your presentation as shown in the following example:

"Ms. J is a 24 y/o G1P1 with an LMP of x/xx/xx presenting with irregular menses."

Thus, the gravida para status and last menstrual period (LMP) are included in the opening statement of your oral presentation. If the patient is postmenopausal, you can say, for example, Mrs. J is a 54 y/o G5P5 LMP >10 years ago who presents with pelvic pain.

IMPORTANT PHYSICAL EXAM FINDINGS AND PHYSIOLOGIC CHANGES DURING PREGNANCY

The list that follows details the physiologic changes that occur during pregnancy.[1]

- Cardiovascular: In normal pregnancies, during the first two trimesters, a physiologic decrease in arterial blood pressure occurs and gradually returns to pregravid numbers. Peripheral vascular resistance decreases. Heart rate increases by about 15 beats per minute during all trimesters. Cardiac output can increase by almost 50% during the third trimester. These changes are responsible for many of the common complaints and physical exam findings in pregnancy, including mild orthostatic hypotension and sometimes presyncope with changing positions; mild dyspnea on exertion, particularly during the third trimester; pedal and leg edema; and even systolic ejection murmurs. Patients who develop syncope, facial edema, unilateral edema, or a diastolic heart murmur should be evaluated expeditiously.

- Hematocrit and hemomglobin: Physiologic declines in hemoglobin and hematocrit occur due to increased plasma volume. This is called an *anemia of dilution*, but it is only considered a true anemia if the hemoglobin and hematocrit drop below 11 g/dL and 33%, respectively. A normal singleton pregnancy requires approximately 1 g of iron per day. Remember to look at the whole picture. If a patient has a low hemoglobin or hematocrit at the first prenatal visit, evaluate the other red blood cell parameters. Determine whether any anemia is microcytic, macrocytic, or normocytic. Make sure you screen for possible hemoglopinopathies when appropriate. Please see the section "Anemia" in Chapter 3, Common Disease Entities in Obstetrics, for more information.
- Respiratory: The diaphragm is displaced superiorly during the second half of pregnancy as the uterus enlarges. This change in position causes a physiologic decrease in resting lung volume (functional residual capacity). Women also experience a physiologic hyperventilatory state during pregnancy that causes respiratory alkalosis. Thus, mild shortness of breath is common in pregnancy, but an acute change requires a thorough history and physical exam.
- Insulin and glucose: As the first trimester ends, gluconeogenesis is decreased, glycogen storage and synthesis are increased, and insulin resistance develops.
- Lipids: Fasting triglycerides increase during pregnancy. There is little evidence that testing of lipids during pregnancy is recommended.
- Thyroid: A thyroid mass in any woman needs investigating, as does a goiter. Thyroid-binding globulin is increased during pregnancy. The thyroid gland will increase in volume during pregnancy. Thyroid-stimulating hormone (TSH) followed by T4 if necessary are appropriate tests of thyroid function in pregnancy.
- Skin: A general hyperpigmentation can occur during pregnancy. The areas most commonly affected are the breasts (particularly the areola), the genitalia, the axilla, the inner thighs, and sometimes the neck. Pay attention to diffuse darkening of the skin because it may be a sign of an endocrinopathy, such as Addison's disease.
- Melasma: This refers to the darkening of skin on the face. This can happen during pregnancy and if a woman is using combined contraception (estrogen plus progestin).
- Breasts: Darkening of the areolas can occur during pregnancy. You may see thick, black hair on the nipples/areola. Some women naturally have more body hair. Some women do not pluck every stray hair on their body. Do not assume that every woman with some hair on her breasts is hyperandrogenic. Remember to look at the whole picture.
- Linea nigra: This is the darkening of the linea alba, the cutaneous line that generally runs from the pubic symphysis up to the xiphoid process. Sometimes it is more pronounced from the pubic symphysis to the umbilicus.

Evidence is mixed regarding the pathogenesis of the linea nigra. Some women who are naturally darker in skin tone may have a darker linea alba, so do not make the mistake of thinking that the presence of a linea nigra is proof that a woman is, or has been, pregnant.

- Stretch marks (striae gravidarum): There is no evidence-based prevention or cure.
- Hair: During pregnancy, hair growth may increase. However, postpartum, many women will complain of significant hair loss. This is called *telogen effluvium*, and it is normal. Sometimes hair thickness and texture will return to its state prior to pregnancy, but sometimes it will not.
- Vagina: A bluish/purplish coloration of the vagina due to increased blood flow is called the *Chadwick sign*. Historically, this was an early sign that helped diagnose pregnancy. Increased leukorrhea is common during pregnancy, and some women complain that they have to use pantiliners daily, particularly during the third trimester.
- Cervix: A bluish/purplish coloration of the cervix is called the *Goodell sign*. Historically, it was used as an early indicator of pregnancy. The cervix also becomes more friable as pregnancy progresses. Postcoital spotting or bleeding is common, but be careful to rule out other causes of bleeding in pregnancy as well.
- Sinus and nasal congestion: This is due to the hormonal state of pregnancy, particularly progesterone. Some women report a heightened sense of smell during pregnancy. This heightened sense of smell can lead to food aversions.
- Gums: During pregnancy, gums can bleed easily. Good oral care is important. Patients should still see a dentist during pregnancy, but the dentist or oral surgeon will likely defer any major surgical intervention until after delivery.
- Hemorrhoids: Many pregnant women develop hemorrhoids during pregnancy and delivery. It is important to educate the patients on good hygiene and ways to prevent irritation and worsening of minor external hemorrhoids. However, any patient who presents with rectal bleeding needs to be appropriately examined and referred for a gastrointestinal (GI) check, when appropriate.
- Varicosities: As pregnancy progresses, the pressure from the uterus can cause venous compression, resulting in varicosities of the vulva and lower extremities. Venous compression can also cause pedal edema, particularly during the third trimester. Unilateral lower extremity edema is a deep vein thrombosis until proven otherwise.
- Prolapse: There are different types of pelvic prolapse: uterine, rectal, bladder, and any combination of two or more. For their identification and management, please see the "Pelvic Organ Prolapse" section in Chapter 2, Common Disease Entities in Gynecology.

Presentation of Fetus During Labor

The most common presentation during a normal labor and delivery is vertex, or cephalic, meaning head down. There are different vertex presentations that correspond to the position of the fetal occiput. If the head is not the presenting part, the baby is in a breech presentation (Figure I.10).

> **Clinical Pearl:** Left occiput anterior (LOA) is the most common presentation. Babies who are born with a posterior occiput are sometimes called "sunny side up."

Medication Prescribing in Pregnancy

Over 50% of women are prescribed at least one medication during pregnancy. The most common reasons include antibiotics for sexually transmitted infections, vaginitis, and urinary tract infections; antiemetics; depression; hypertensive disorders of pregnancy; preterm labor; diabetes mellitus; and asthma.[2]

The physiologic changes during pregnancy can affect pharmacokinetics and pharmacodynamics.[3]

Pharmacokinetics involve drug absorption, distribution, metabolism, and excretion. *Pharmacodynamics* involves the effects of the drug on the body. During pregnancy, the effect of the drug on the fetus must be considered at all times.

During the first trimester while the fetus is still developing, exposure to drugs can cause abnormalities in fetal development (Table I.1). Some women will present for their initial prenatal visit at 10 or 12 weeks, and history reveals that they had taken a drug, either prescribed or illicit, before they even knew they were pregnant. If the drug is known to cause harm to the developing fetus, these women need to be counseled and evaluated very closely, preferably with maternal–fetal medicine consultation. However, as the fetus continues to develop during the second and third trimesters, exposures during these times can also exert an adverse effect.

Teratogenicity is the term that is used to describe the effect of an exposure on the fetus. Remember that there are other teratogens besides drugs, including some infectious agents, such as the TORCH group. TORCH stands for **t**oxoplasmosis, **o**thers, **r**ubella, **c**ytomegalovirus, and **h**erpes. There are several prescribed drugs that are known teratogens (Table I.1). Certain antiseizure drugs, retinoids, lithium, and angiotensin II receptor antagonists are known to be teratogenic. Alcohol is also teratogenic.

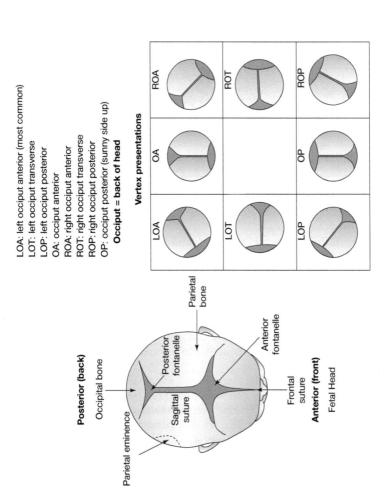

LOA: left occiput anterior (most common)
LOT: left occiput transverse
LOP: left occiput posterior
OA: occiput anterior
ROA: right occiput anterior
ROT: right occiput transverse
ROP: right occiput posterior
OP: occiput posterior (sunny side up)
Occiput = back of head

Vertex presentations

LOA	OA	ROA
LOT		ROT
LOP	OP	ROP

Posterior (back)

Occipital bone

Posterior fontanelle

Parietal eminence

Sagittal suture

Parietal bone

Anterior fontanelle

Frontal suture

Anterior (front)

Fetal Head

FIGURE 1.10 Fetal head and vertex presentations.

TABLE I.1 Prescription Medications Known to Cause Harm in the Developing Fetus

Medication	Associated Effects
Androgenic progestins	Masculinization of female fetus
Alcohol	Fetal alcohol syndrome: mental retardation/developmental delays, microcephaly, ocular abnormalities, short palpebral fissures, intrauterine growth restriction, congenital heart disease
Lithium	Cardiovascular malformations
Phenytoin	Microcephaly, intrauterine growth restriction, inner epicanthal folds, eyelid ptosis, mental retardation/developmental delays, broadened and depressed nasal bridge, phalangeal hypoplasia
Retinoids (and excessive vitamin A)	Neural tube defects
Tetracycline	Enamel hypoplasia, stained teeth
Valproic acid	Flattened nasal bridge, microstomia, neural tube defects

CLINICAL PEARL: Utilize an appropriate and current drug reference that includes over-the-counter and herbal products to provide information on the safety of products patients may ingest.

One of the most important pieces of information you need to know before prescribing any medication is whether that medication can cross the placenta. Heparins, for example, do not cross the placenta and, as such, are considered safe in pregnancy.

Some of the common physiologic changes that are associated with changes in drug absorption and excretion include nausea and vomiting in early pregnancy, an increase in renal perfusion resulting in an increased drug clearance, and changes in hepatic drug clearance. The increase in plasma volume and pregnancy hormone effects on the liver also affect the way a drug is absorbed, metabolized, distributed, and excreted.

The Food and Drug Administration changed the Pregnancy Categories for drugs from A, B, C, D, and X to a narrative that describes the current state of the evidence regarding the drug and its effect during pregnancy and lactation. Please refer to the article by Watkins and Archambault[4] for a review of the changes.

What Previous Physician Assistant Students Wish They Knew Before This Rotation

Many students say that there are certain things they wish they knew before their OB/GYN rotation. Here are a few items mentioned by former students:

- Trimesters (tests performed, number of weeks, how the mother is typically feeling/body changes)
- Stages of delivery
- Abnormal uterine bleeding causes based on age
- Clinical decision-making with Pap testing and human papillomavirus (HPV) results
- Progestin versus combined oral contraceptive pills (OCPs)
- Polycystic ovarian syndrome
- Menstrual cycle (main hormone changes and what they mean)
- Prenatal testing options: timing, what they test for, sensitivity, specificity
- When patients should go to the hospital for labor
- Labor complications
- When to induce labor
- Preeclampsia/eclampsia
- Placenta previa/accreta: what it is, how to diagnose
- Explaining different types of spontaneous abortions, how to monitor, who gets medications, and who gets surgery
- Major labor complications (shoulder dystocia, postpartum hemorrhage)
- Tips for how to do a pelvic exam
- The components of the gynecologic exam
- Conditions that can affect the fetus in utero, such as causes and treatment of polyhydramnios or oligohydramnios, as well as causes of intrauterine growth restriction (IUGR)
- Causes and treatment of postpartum hemorrhage
- Infertility causes, the workup of infertility

Pertinent Specialty-Specific Physical Exams

New obstetric patients and well-woman exam patients must have a complete physical exam, including head, ears, eyes, nose, and throat (HEENT) and the cardiopulmonary system. It is easy to just perform a breast exam and a pelvic exam. Please do not take shortcuts. If you think you hear something or see something abnormal, tell your preceptor. Malignant melanomas, heart murmurs, and thyroid masses that were previously undiagnosed may be found during a physical examination on a patient being seen for a new obstetric visit or well-woman exam.

> **CLINICAL PEARL:** Many women use their OB/GYN providers as their primary care providers. The Pap test visit may be their only opportunity for a complete physical examination.

PELVIC EXAM

Always make sure you have a chaperone in the room with you. The chaperone must be another employee in the clinic or office. You cannot use a family member to be the chaperone, and if you are a male physician assistant (PA) student, you must have a female chaperone present. If the patient does not speak English, you must use a translator. A family member cannot serve as a translator.

External Inspection

The first part of the pelvic examination consists of inspecting the vulva; the Bartholin glands, the urethra, the Skene's glands (collectively referred to as BUS); the perineum; the anus; and the introitus, or opening of the vagina. There are four steps to prepare for the exam.

1. Make sure you have a light source that works. It can be frustrating to have the patient ready to go and realize that the light source has been unplugged.
2. Make sure the patient's legs are in the heel rests and wide enough for you to visualize the anatomy and perform the examination.
3. Ask the patient to slide all the way down to the end of the table so that the buttocks are right at the bottom of the table. Reassure the patient that you will make sure she does not fall.
4. Check the positioning of the lap sheet. You want to ensure adequate coverage yet enough exposure for you to do what you need to do.

> **CLINICAL PEARL:** Be absolutely sure you have everything you need before beginning the exam. For example, if the patient is bleeding, have extra absorbent pads available.

While inspecting, do not be afraid to move the vulva and excess skin folds out of the way, but make sure you tell the patient that you are going to be examining her and that she is going to feel your hand touching her. Some women have thicker or longer vulva that can make visualization difficult. Be sure to inspect completely. You may find malignant melanomas of the vulva and inner thighs by being very diligent with the examination technique (Figure I.11).

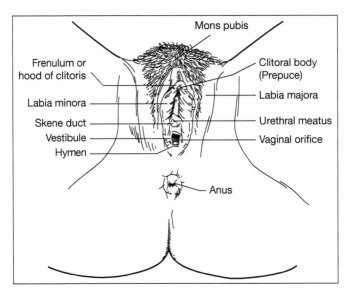

Figure I.11 External female genitalia.
Source: From Secor RM, Fantasia HC. *Fast Facts About the Gynecologic Exam.* 2nd ed. New York, NY: Springer Publishing Company;2018:28.

The Speculum Exam

The second part of the pelvic exam involves inserting a speculum into the vagina to visualize the vaginal walls and the cervix. This is a skill that requires practice. Here are a few pearls to help you.

1. Hold the speculum with your dominant hand. Make sure it is opening and closing normally before you insert it. Sometimes the less expensive plastic models will have defects that you want to identify prior to insertion.
2. Approach the introitus slowly, holding the speculum at about a 30- to 45-degree angle. When you make initial contact, the speculum should be at the posterior vaginal wall. Avoid entering the vagina with anterior pressure because you will hit the clitoris and urethra, causing discomfort. The patient will reflexively tense up, making full insertion of the speculum difficult.
3. While continuing to apply posterior pressure with the speculum, slowly insert and open the speculum with a slight rotation, allowing the speculum to be open enough to visualize the cervix.
4. Once you have the cervix in view, rotate the speculum enough to bring it to a perpendicular position with the handle at the bottom.
5. Lock the speculum and ask the patient whether she is doing all right before you begin to take any specimens, such as cultures, polymerase chain reactions (PCRs), or Pap tests.

6. Always tell the patient what you are going to do before you do it.
7. When you have completed the specimen retrieval, tell the patient you are done and that you are now going to remove the speculum.
8. DO NOT begin to remove the speculum at this point. You must first completely unlock the speculum so that it starts to narrow. Once it has been unlocked, retract the speculum a few centimeters so that the cervix falls out of view. Then begin to remove the speculum with downward pressure to avoid the clitoris or urethra.
9. Be calm and be deliberate, but do not take too long. The patient is in a vulnerable position that is uncomfortable.
10. Do not whisper to your medical assistant or nurse while performing a pelvic exam.

The Bimanual Exam

The bimanual exam is performed after the speculum exam. You will insert two fingers (the second and third digits) of your dominant hand into the vagina, and use your other hand to palpate the uterus and adnexa. This can be uncomfortable for the patient, so it is important to tell the patient everything you are doing.

There are several reasons why a bimanual exam is performed. It allows the examiner to palpate the uterus and adnexa to assess for masses, tenderness, and mobility (Figure I.12). A normal nongravid uterus is about the size of a fist. Normally, the ovaries are about 3 to 5 cm. You may not palpate very many ovaries during your clinical rotation. The first reason is that sometimes the ovaries lay deeper, or more posteriorly, in the pelvis. The second reason is that if there is significant abdominal adiposity, it can be difficult to palpate through the adipose layer (and the musculature as well).

A few pearls for performing the bimanual exam:

1. Make sure you put a little bit of lubricant on your fingers before you insert them into the vagina.
2. As when you inserted the speculum, apply posterior pressure while inserting to avoid the clitoris and urethra.
3. Once you have inserted your fingers, find the cervix. In a nongravid patient, its consistency is similar to the end of your nose.
4. When the cervix has been located, push caudally, in a gentle motion, and use your nondominant hand to find the fundus of the uterus. An important physical exam finding during the bimanual is assessing whether or not the uterus is mobile.
5. Palpate along the top of the fundus to assess for shape and size. If you feel any lumps, this could be a fibroid. Depending on where the ovaries lie, sometimes an ovarian cyst will feel as if it is part of the uterus. You will have to obtain an ultrasound to further investigate any abnormal masses on the bimanual exam.

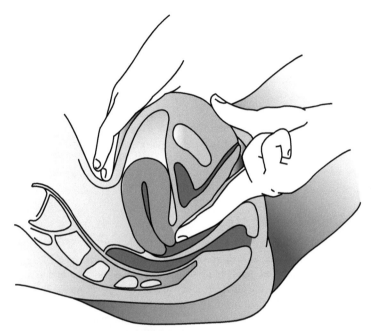

Figure I.12   Bimanual examination: Palpation of an anteverted uterus.
The examiner is unable to palpate the body or fundus of the uterus between the vaginal and abdominal examination fingers.

6. Some women experience discomfort during the bimanual exam, particularly when you push on the cervix. It is important to differentiate normal discomfort from a true "chandelier sign," or cervical motion tenderness, as these findings can indicate pelvic inflammatory disease. Sometimes women with endometriosis or adenomyosis will have discomfort or pain with cervical motion. You must look at the whole picture.

> **Clinical Pearl:** Patients who have endured sexual abuse can have difficulty with a pelvic examination. Never force an exam, and always provide emotional support.

Breast Exam

With the patient in the supine position, expose one breast at a time. Pay attention to the skin, contour, presence of scars or lesions, nipple inversion or eversion, and any other visual abnormalities. When you begin palpating, use the tips of two fingers and methodically palpate the entire breast, including the tail. If a patient is presenting with a possible breast mass, you must also inspect the breasts while the patient is sitting, and you must palpate for axillary and infra- and supraclavicular lymphadenopathy. If the patient is complaining of nipple discharge, it may be helpful to have the patient attempt expression of fluid.

> **CLINICAL PEARL:** It is not uncommon for one breast to be larger than the other. If the patient is not bothered, it is unnecessary to address this as a problem.

OBSTETRIC CHECKS

Fetal Heart Tones

Place some ultrasound gel on the abdomen. Turn on the handheld Doppler and place it on the gel. Apply minimal pressure and do not be afraid to move the Doppler around the abdomen. Be patient. Fetal heart tones (FHTs) can generally be heard beginning at 10 weeks, but in some obese women, it may be difficult. Always consider the gestational age of the pregnancy so that you can visualize or palpate the fundus and know that you will have to auscultate well below the fundus. Normal FHTs are anywhere between 120 and 160 beats per minute.[5]

> **CLINICAL PEARL:** If you cannot find the FHTs with the Doppler, do not alarm the patient. Ask someone more experienced to help you.

Fundal Height

In singleton pregnancies, palpating fundal height through the abdomen can begin after 20 weeks. Around 20 weeks, the fundus is at the level of the umbilicus. You will need a tape measure that has centimeter markings. First, palpate the symphysis pubis. Hold the end of the tape measure beginning at the symphysis pubis and extend the tape measure to the fundus, or the top of the uterus. After 20 weeks, the height of the fundus should equal, plus or minus 2 cm, the gestational age of the pregnancy (Figure I.13).

> **CLINICAL PEARL:** Measuring the fundal height on an obese patient with a large pannus can be difficult. You may have to ask her to lift the pannus toward her head so you can measure.

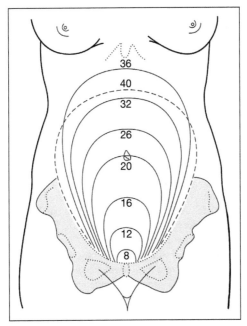

FIGURE I.13   Uterine fundal height.
Source: From Carcio HA, Secor RM. *Advanced Health Assessment of Women: Clinical Skills and Procedures.* 4th ed. New York, NY: Springer Publishing Company; 2019:136.

CERVICAL CHECKS

Checking the cervix for dilation and effacement should not be regularly performed prior to 36 weeks unless the patient has specific complaints that may indicate preterm labor. However, if a patient has symptoms of preterm labor, you do not immediately perform a cervical check (see the section "Preterm Labor" in Chapter 3, Common Disease Entities in Obstetrics). Routine cervical checks on a term patient are typically done weekly (from 36 weeks until delivery). The idea is to get a sense of the position of the fetus, the station, and the dilation and effacement of the cervix.

CLINICAL PEARL: Students can become frustrated with cervical checks for effacement and dilation. This skill is learned through repetition. Do not be disappointed if you are not correct with your initial estimates. The more cervixes you palpate, the better you will become at assessing dilation and effacement.

USE OF INTERPROFESSIONAL CONSULTATIONS

Referrals to urogynecological physical therapists can be helpful when a woman is experiencing urinary incontinence and early pelvic organ prolapse. The therapist can teach the patient how to perform Kegel exercises appropriately by using specific devices that allow the patient to receive immediate feedback on the strength and duration of pelvic floor contractions.

There may be times when you identify a patient who is a victim of domestic violence, human trafficking, or a perpetrator of child abuse or neglect. We are mandated reporters, so you must be prepared to talk to your preceptor about your concerns before the patient leaves the office. Due to the potential legal ramifications, your preceptor should perform the physical exam and document appropriately. Domestic violence and human trafficking laws may vary by state, so your preceptor may be the one most familiar with those laws, particularly if you are at a rotation out of state.

Familiarize yourself with the appropriate local agency to which to refer. Most communities will have a local women's shelter for victims of domestic abuse. Women's shelters provide emergency housing, counseling, and advocacy.

Human-trafficking victims may present with recurrent sexually transmitted diseases, recurrent unwanted pregnancies, depression/anxiety, and/or physical trauma. Most victims of human trafficking will present with their captor, who speaks for them. Pay attention to the nonverbal communication and whether the woman is allowed to speak for herself. For more information on antihuman trafficking, call the National Human Trafficking Hotline at 1 (888) 373-7888.

Many times the woman will not want to immediately report the abuse to local law enforcement, but you should always ask. If she wants to speak to law enforcement, tell your preceptor right away so that the appropriate chain of events occurs. If she does not want to report the abuse, give her the contact information for the shelters that serve the community.

If you suspect child abuse or neglect, notify your preceptor and be prepared to file with local child protective services. Some examples of child abuse or neglect that you may encounter in an OB/GYN setting include the following:

1. A child who is inappropriately dressed for the weather (e.g., no shoes or socks during colder months).
2. A child who is unkempt.
3. The patient tells you about illicit drug use that is occurring at her place of residence and that there are children living there.

CLINICAL PEARL: When suspicious of abuse, notify your preceptor immediately.

CONFIDENTIALITY PRACTICES AND ETHICS

Women generally do not like going to the OB/GYN office. The lithotomy position is uncomfortable and places women in a vulnerable position. It is difficult for some women to talk about the intimate details of their lives with a stranger, so do not take it personally if the patient refuses to let you take the history or perform the physical exam.

You are going to be privy to information that can be shocking and distressing. It is imperative that you learn how not to respond with shock, horror, judgment, or even revulsion. You will hear about sexual practices that may not align with your own idea of "normal." You will hear about choices women make that may not align with your own set of values. Your job is to learn from each of these women. Learn about their lives, their challenges, and meet them wherever they may be. Sometimes, the most therapeutic act is to simply listen.

Never discuss your own issues. If a woman is experiencing a miscarriage, and you or your partner had one also, please do not share that with the patient. Let each patient's experience be her experience. It is never about you.

Never discuss any patient issue with anyone outside of the practice setting and only when absolutely necessary, such as when you present to your preceptor. Be mindful of where you present as well. Avoid conversations in the hallway where others can overhear you and your preceptor. As is true in any practice setting, the Health Insurance Portability and Accountability Act (HIPAA) applies to all encounters, so be careful what you say outside of the exam rooms. Finally, never post anything on social media regarding your rotation.

SAMPLE DOCUMENTATION

Sample documentation of a gynecologic exam (considering everything is normal)

Breasts: Symmetrical, no skin dimpling or lesions visualized, nipples are everted bilaterally. No dominant masses palpated, no nipple discharge expressed, and no axillary lymphadenopathy palpated.

Pelvic: Patient was in lithotomy position with feet in stirrups, Ms. Smith, MA, was present. Vulva has no lesions, erythema, or hypopigmentation. BUS without lesions or masses. Anus without lesions, external hemorrhoids, or fissures. Introitus without lesions. Speculum inserted without difficulty and cervix visualized. Ectropion present but no erythema, lesions, bleeding, or friability of the cervix. The cervix is long and closed. Pap test obtained. Speculum removed without difficulty. Bimanual exam revealed uterus of normal size, shape, and consistency, no cervical motion tenderness, adnexa without masses or tenderness palpated.

REFERENCES

1. Koos BJ, Hobel CJ. Maternal physiologic and immunologic adaptation to pregnancy. In: Hacker N, Gambone J, Hobel C, eds. *Hacker & Moore's Essentials of Obstetrics and Gynecology*. 6th ed. Philadelphia, PA: Elsevier; 2016:61–75.

2. Chambers CD, Polifka JE, Friedman JM. Drug safety in pregnant women and their babies: ignorance not bliss. *Clin Pharmacol Ther*. 2008;83(1):181–183. doi:10.1038/sj.clpt.6100448.

3. Zhao Y, Hebert MF, Venkataramanan R. Basic obstetric pharmacology. *Semin Perinatol*. 2014;38(8):475–486. doi:10.1053/j.semperi.2014.08.011

4. Watkins EJ, Archambault M. Understanding the new pregnancy and lactation drug labeling. *JAAPA*. 2016;29(2):50–52. doi:10.1097/01.JAA.0000475474.25004.cf

5. Kilpatrick SJ, Papile L-A, Macones GA, eds. *Guidelines for Perinatal Care*. 8th ed. Elk Grove, IL: American Academy of Pediatrics; Washington, DC: American College of Obstetricians and Gynecologists; 2017.

1

Common Presentations in Obstetrics and Gynecology

Introduction

The women's health OB/GYN clinical rotation is an opportunity for you to learn about common, and sometimes uncommon, gynecologic and obstetric conditions. When a patient presents with a chief complaint, you should immediately begin to think about the differential diagnosis, but it is helpful to categorize patients as premenopausal or postmenopausal as soon as you obtain the chief complaint. The differential diagnosis for vaginal bleeding in a 20-year-old will be very different than that in a 60-year-old.

Always consider the possible diagnoses that can be deadly for a patient. For a patient with vaginal discharge, there are not many etiologies than can cause imminent death, but for a patient with irregular vaginal bleeding, an ectopic pregnancy or endometrial cancer can most certainly cause death. It is also a good rule of thumb to consider all women of reproductive age (generally between the ages of 12 and 45) to be pregnant until proven otherwise.

When presented with a chief complaint in a nonpregnant patient, remember that sometimes what the patient tells the medical assistant or nurse will not be what actually brings the patient in to be seen. You may want to start by knocking on the door, entering once permission has been given, introducing yourself with your name (and stating that you are a physician assistant [PA] student), and then asking, "What can I help you with today?" It can be awkward if you walk in and state, "I understand that you have been having some pelvic pain" when in reality, the patient wanted to tell you about something unrelated to the generic chief complaint she told the receptionist or medical assistant or nurse. Many women will not want to tell anyone else about her vaginal discharge or sexual issue.

Once you have established what the actual chief complaint is, begin formulating your differential diagnosis. What questions will help you rule in or rule out certain diseases? Often the person who rooms the patient will have asked about the patient's last menstrual period (LMP), but it is always a good idea to verify this with the patient.

Use whichever mnemonic is most helpful regarding taking the history and developing a history of present illness (HPI). Two of the most common are OLDCARTS (onset, location, duration, character, aggravating factors, relieving factors, timing, severity) and OPQRST (onset, provoking/alleviating factors, quality, radiation, severity, timing).

Once you have begun to list a few common diagnoses for the chief complaint, you may want to employ another mnemonic to help you identify other possibilities and create a broad differential diagnosis list. One example is VINDICATE.

- V—Vascular
- I—Inflammatory
- N—Neoplastic
- D—Degenerative/deficiency
- I—Idiopathic, intoxication
- C—Congenital
- A—Autoimmune/allergic
- T—Traumatic
- E—Endocrine

Summarize the pertinent negative and positive data. At this point, you can begin formulating a working differential diagnosis. Try to rank your diagnoses by order of most likely to least likely. It can be fun as a student to chase a zebra, but remember, when you hear hoof beats, they are usually caused by a horse. However, always be mindful of diagnoses that are associated with a high risk of mortality.

Next, think about what physical examination findings and ancillary testing will help you rule in and rule out your diagnoses. For example, patients who present with vaginal discharge will need to have a pelvic exam with a wet mount and/or a polymerase chain reaction (PCR) analysis. Think about what other ancillary testing might be necessary to help you with your diagnosis. What can be accomplished today? Will you need to schedule the patient for an ultrasound or order labs?

Begin to think about your care plan. This can be tricky if you are waiting on labs or an ultrasound report. Always make sure the patient understands the plan and that you have provided appropriate documentation that outlines the care plan. The plan must always contain specific instructions about when to return and under what conditions the patient should go to the ED or labor and delivery.

Five of the most common chief complaints you are likely to encounter in an outpatient OB/GYN setting include irregular menses, missed menses, pelvic pain, prenatal visits, and vaginal discharge. For more information on specific disease entities, please refer to Chapters 1 to 3.

Irregular Menses/Abnormal Uterine Bleeding

Menorrhagia, or heavy menstrual bleeding, is bleeding that lasts more than 7 days per cycle, and/or in which more than 80 mL of vaginal blood is sloughed. Menometrorrhagia, or intermenstrual bleeding, is greater than 80 mL of blood loss at irregular intervals.[1]

The menstrual cycle consists of three phases: the follicular phase, ovulatory phase, and the luteal phase (early and late). Each phase is the result of a complex interaction among the hypothalamus, the anterior pituitary, the ovaries, and the endometrium. The average duration of menstrual bleeding is 5 days, and cycle length is 28 days.

"Normal" bleeding pattern:

- 5 days of bleeding
- Heaviest bleeding on day 2
- ~30 mL of blood loss total
- Occurs every 28 days

Differential Diagnosis

The first step in formulating your differential diagnosis is to determine whether the patient is pre- or postmenopausal. In a postmenopausal woman, vaginal bleeding is uterine cancer until proven otherwise. In premenopausal women, particularly if obese, the most common diagnosis is anovulation/oligo-ovulation. American College of Obstetricians and Gynecologists (ACOG) suggests the use of the mnemonic PALM-COEIN to help guide the differential diagnosis. Abnormal uterine bleeding (AUB) is classified using the PALM-COEIN system (Table 1.1). PALM is the acronym for the structural causes of AUB, which stands for polyp, adenomyosis, leiomyoma, malignancy and hyperplasia. COEIN is the acronym for the nonstructural causes of AUB, which stands for coagulopathy, ovulatory dysfunction, endometrial, iatrogenic, and not otherwise classified.

TABLE 1.1 Abnormal Uterine Bleeding Differential Diagnosis Mnemonic: PALM-COEIN

PALM (Structural)	COEIN (Nonstructural)
Polyp	Coagulopathy
Adenomyosis	Ovarian
Leiomyoma	Endometrial
Malignancy	Iatrogenic
	Not yet classified

A more comprehensive differential diagnosis includes iatrogenic, blood dyscrasias, infection, malignancy, benign growths, and systemic disease (Table 1.2). It is also important to consider possible trauma, which can be ruled out when performing a pelvic examination. Often, the diagnosis is one of exclusion.

TABLE 1.2 Differential Diagnosis of Abnormal Uterine Bleeding

Category	Examples
Iatrogenic	IUS
	Oral contraceptive pills (both combination of estrogen and progestin, and progestin alone)
	Other hormonal contraception (such as patches, rings, injections, and implants
	Antiplatelet medications
	Anticoagulant medications
Hematologic	Von Willebrand disease
	Leukemia
	Thrombocytopenia
Infection	Cervicitis
	Pelvic inflammatory disease
	Endometritis
Malignancy	Cervical cancer
	Uterine cancer
	Endometrial hyperplasia with atypia
Benign growths	Leiomyoma
	Endometrial hyperplasia without atypia
	Uterine and endocervical polyps
	Adenomyosis
Systemic disease	Thyroid disease
	Renal disease
	Liver disease
	Polycystic ovarian syndrome

IUS, intrauterine system.

History

Taking a thorough history is still the cornerstone of medical practice. Consider the differential diagnoses when asking questions relevant to your history of present illness (HPI) so that you can begin to rank the possible etiologies. Do not forget to ask whether this has ever happened before, and if so, what helped or did not help.

- Onset, duration, and timing: If the bleeding occurs cyclically, with each menses, you can probably eliminate trauma from your differential list. Ask the patient to describe how many pads or tampons she is using each day. For how many days does the bleeding last? Did the irregular bleeding start once the patient began taking a new medication? Did the patient recently have an IUS inserted?

> **CLINICAL PEARL:** Postmenopausal bleeding is endometrial cancer until proven otherwise.

- Provoking/alleviating factors: Ask the patient whether sexual intercourse causes or increases bleeding. Often, NSAIDs will alleviate mild dysmenorrhea and heavier bleeding when taken at the onset of symptoms.

> **CLINICAL PEARL:** Postcoital bleeding is usually due to a benign polyp or cervicitis. It can also occur in pregnancy, so make sure the patient is not pregnant.

- Severity: Quantify the blood loss by asking how many pads and/or tampons the patient uses in a day.

> **CLINICAL PEARL:** On average, women will lose about 30 mL of blood during each cycle. Changing pads/tampons more than once every hour due to saturation for more than a day is likely not normal. Ask the patient whether she has to wake up during the night to change pads/tampons, and if she soaks through clothing. Also remember that the heaviest days of bleeding are usually days 1 and 2.

- Associated symptoms: Ask the patient about pain with bleeding. Be sure to assess whether the patient is experiencing any fatigue, fever, bleeding from other locations (such as gums), easy bruisability, skin changes, tachycardia, presyncope or syncope, changes in appetite, unintentional weight changes, and abdominal or pelvic bloating.

> **CLINICAL PEARL:** Patients who present with menorrhagia/heavy menstrual bleeding and have any signs of volume compromise or severe anemia need to be managed emergently.

Past Medical History and Review of Symptoms Specific to Complaint

- OB/GYN: Always obtain the patient's gravida and para status and use of contraception. Chronic unintentional anovulation is a risk factor for endometrial cancer. Patients with a history of estrogen positive breast cancer who take a selective estrogen receptor modulator (SERM) are at a slightly increased risk of endometrial hyperplasia/cancer.

> **CLINICAL PEARL:** Irregular bleeding in a patient with a positive pregnancy test and no confirmation of an intrauterine pregnancy is an ectopic until proven otherwise.

- Urinary: Ask about hematuria, frequency, urgency, incontinence, and difficulty emptying the bladder.

> **CLINICAL PEARL:** Leiomyoma can cause irregular bleeding and, depending on where the fibroid is located, can cause a "mass effect" that may present as urinary problems.

- Endocrine: Ask about a history of thyroid disorders, diabetes, and insulin resistance. Patients who are obese are at risk for endometrial hyperplasia and endometrial cancer.

> **CLINICAL PEARL:** Patients with thyroid abnormalities can present with irregular menses, and patients with polycystic ovarian syndrome will usually present with oligomenorrhea/infrequent menses.

- GI: Ask whether the patient has constipation or diarrhea; abdominal pain; dyspepsia; bleeding with bowel movements; changes with bowel movements, including frequency, shape, and color of stool; changes in appetite; and nausea and vomiting.

> **CLINICAL PEARL:** Leiomyoma can cause heavy menses, and, depending on the size and position of the fibroid, can affect bowel habits.

- Hematologic: Ask the patient about a history of blood dyscrasias and whether the patient takes anticoagulants or antiplatelet medications. It is important to also assess hypercoagulable risk factors because the treatment of heavy menstrual bleeding/menorrhagia, in the absence of endometrial cancer or pregnancy, is often estrogen administration.

> **CLINICAL PEARL:** Young women with irregular menses, particularly heavy menstrual bleeding, can have a bleeding problem, such as Von Willebrand disease.

Social History

Ask about sexual practices, possible trauma, and if the patient uses illicit drugs or tobacco.

Physical Examination

Many women will not want you to perform a pelvic exam while they are bleeding. Please reassure your patient that it is necessary, and that you will take every precaution to ensure your patient is as comfortable as you can allow. It is important to make sure you locate from where the bleeding is coming.

Ask your patient whether she is currently wearing a tampon. If so, have her remove it prior to the examination. If using a pad, ask her whether she has a fresh pad to use once the exam is over. If not, be prepared to offer one to the patient at the end of your exam.

Perhaps most important, place a Chux under the patient's buttocks and if necessary, another one on the footstool of the examination table. Sometimes the bleeding is so heavy that it will be necessary to place a Chux between you and the trash container. Remember that when you remove the speculum from the patient's vagina, there can be a lot of blood. You do not want to spill the blood on yourself or on the floor. Be prepared to have the garbage close by. Sometimes it is also necessary to have an extra Chux on which to place the speculum once it has been removed from the vagina prior to placing it in the trash.

It can be difficult to adequately visualize the cervix when there is significant bleeding. You must be prepared to place gauze held by a ring forceps or several large cotton swabs in the vagina and around the cervix to absorb some of the blood. You can easily miss a cervical carcinoma, which can bleed quite profusely when advanced, by not visualizing the cervix. See Table 1.3 for physical examination findings that correlate with clinical conditions.

> **CLINICAL PEARL:** Never wear open-toe shoes to any of your clinical rotations. In OB/GYN, you will likely end up with urine and/or blood on your shoes, so invest in a good pair of healthcare professional waterproof clogs or shoes.

TABLE 1.3 Correlating Physical Exam Findings With Pathologic Conditions

Body or Organ System	Physical Exam Finding	Associated Clinical Condition
General appearance	Fatigued	Hypothyroidism, anemia
Vital signs	Tachycardia	Anemia, acute blood loss
	Hypotension	Acute blood loss
Skin	Pallor	Anemia
	Petechiae, purpura	Thrombocytopenia, ESRD
	Palmar erythema, jaundice, spider angiomas	Liver disease
Abdomen	Ascites, distention	Liver disease, malignancy
	Caput medusae	Liver disease
Vulva and perineum	Lacerations	Trauma
Vagina	Lacerations, hematoma	Trauma
	Foreign object	Foreign object
	Decreased rugae	Vulvovaginal atrophy
Cervix	Endocervical polyp	Endocervical polyp
	Friability	Cervicitis, cervical cancer
	IUS string	IUS in situ
Adnexa	Mass	Malignancy
Uterus	Masses	Leiomyoma
	Enlargement	Leiomyoma, adenomyosis, pregnancy
	Fixed, immobile	Malignancy

ESRD, end-stage renal disease; IUS, intrauterine system.

Diagnostic Plan

Pregnancy must be ruled out in all patients with irregular bleeding. A postmenopausal woman with vaginal bleeding has uterine cancer until proven otherwise.

If a patient is deemed to be hemodynamically unstable, the goal is to stabilize the patient utilizing basic life-support principles. As such, patients who present to the outpatient setting with heavy menstrual bleeding/menorrhagia and are deemed unstable require prompt referral to an ED via emergency medical transport. If the patient is hemodynamically stable, the workup should include basic and more invasive testing, as necessary.

- Human chorionic gonadotropic assay: All patients of reproductive age with a uterus must have a pregnancy test.
  - Evaluate for pregnancy.
- Complete blood count (CBC) with platelets will help to quantify blood loss, but remember that in acute blood loss, the hemoglobin and hematocrit may not have yet changed.
  - Evaluate for presence and severity of anemia, infection, thrombocytopenia.

Further laboratory testing based upon history and physical examination:

- Iron studies are needed if the patient has a microcytic anemia
  - Evaluate for iron deficiency anemia
- Coagulation panel: Prothrombin time (PT), activated partial thromboplastin time (aPTT), bleeding time, fibrinogen
  - Evaluate for coagulopathy
- Liver enzymes: Alanine aminotransferase (ALT) and aspartate aminotransferase (AST)
  - Evaluate for underlying liver disease that can affect estrogen metabolism
- Von Willebrand factor ([vWF] VIII coagulant activity, ristocetin cofactor activity, vWF antigen; sometimes available as a VW panel) and factor XI: generally limited to adolescent/younger patients
  - Evaluate for the presence of a bleeding disorder
- Thyroid function tests: Thyroid-stimulating hormone (TSH)and free T4
  - Evaluate for underlying thyroid disease
- Prolactin: Hyperprolactinemia can cause ovulatory dysfunction
  - Evaluate for evidence of a pituitary adenoma and/or hyperprolactinemia

Other diagnostic modalities that should be considered include pelvic sonography, endometrial biopsy, cervical cytology (Pap testing) per current guidelines; and hysteroscopy, hysterosonography, and dilation and curettage, depending on the clinical picture. See Table 1.4 for correlations among diagnostic modalities, positive findings, and clinical conditions.

TABLE 1.4 Diagnostic Modalities for Abnormal Uterine Bleeding

Diagnostic Modality	Positive Findings	Common Clinical Condition
Pelvic ultrasonography	Adnexal mass	Ovarian cyst(s), neoplasia
	Uterine mass	Leiomyoma, adenomyosis
	Thickened endometrium	Endometrial hyperplasia[a]

(*continued*)

TABLE **1.4** Diagnostic Modalities for Abnormal Uterine Bleeding (*continued*)

Diagnostic Modality	Positive Findings	Common Clinical Condition
Endometrial biopsy	Endometrial hyperplasia	Premalignant or malignant endometrial neoplasia
Cervical cytology	High-grade lesion	Cervical dysplasia or carcinoma[b]
Hysteroscopy	Proliferative endometrium	Premalignant or malignant endometrial neoplasia
	Polyp	Endometrial polyp
	Leiomyoma	Submucosal leiomyoma
Hysterosonography	Diffuse thickening, focal thickening	Endometrial hyperplasia, endometrial cancer, endometrial polyp, submucosal leiomyoma
Dilation and curettage	Endometrial hyperplasia	Premalignant or malignant endometrial neoplasia

[a] Endometrial thickness should be correlated with the patient's menstrual cycle.
[b] Cytology is a screening test; must perform a biopsy via colposcopy for definitive diagnosis.

Initial Management

- The management of abnormal uterine bleeding will depend on the presence or absence of underlying pathology.
- Emergency management of heavy menstrual bleeding that causes volume compromise includes intravenous conjugated equine estrogens 25 mg every 4 to 6 hours for 24 hours (if no contraindications exist) or tranexamic acid 1.3 g orally or 10 mg/kg for a maximum dose of 600 mg, with fluid support.
- If patients have contraindications for estrogen and tranexamic acid, a 26F Foley catheter with 30 mL of saline can be placed in the uterus for uterine tamponade.
- Heavy menstrual bleeding/menorrhagia that causes a significant decrease in hemoglobin/hematocrit should be assessed for possible blood and clotting factor replacement.
- Once uterine or cervical malignancy and pregnancy have been ruled out, and the patient is hemodynamically stable, expectant management may be considered.
- Other treatment options include oral tranexamic acid, estrogen and progestin combinations, progestin-secreting IUSs, uterine artery embolization, and, for patients who either do not respond to, have a contraindication for hormone use, and who are certain they will not desire future pregnancy, endometrial ablation can be considered, but is not considered first-line therapy.

- Endometrial ablation is the preferred treatment modality prior to hysterectomy due to decreased morbidity.
- Adolescents without contraindications should be offered combination hormonal contraceptives or a progestin-secreting IUS for the management of irregular menstrual bleeding.
- Hysterectomy is reserved for patients in whom a malignancy has been identified or who have had failed other interventions.

> **CLINICAL PEARL:** Women with risk factors for endometrial cancer (obesity, age greater than 45 years, chronic anovulation or oligo-ovulation) should undergo endometrial sampling as soon as possible.

Key Points . . .

- Assess the patient for hemodynamic compromise. Certain gynecologic and obstetrical disorders can cause hemorrhage and hemodynamic collapse.
- Uterine bleeding in a postmenopausal woman is endometrial cancer until proven otherwise.
- A reproductive-aged patient with irregular uterine bleeding must be ruled out for pregnancy.
- An appropriate focused history and physical exam will help you narrow your differential diagnosis.

REFERENCE

1. American College of Obstetricians and Gynecologists. ACOG Committee Opinion No. 557: management of acute abnormal uterine bleeding in nonpregnant reproductive-aged women. *Obstet Gynecol.* 2013;121:891–896. doi:10.1097/01.AOG.0000428646.67925.9a. Reaffirmed 2019.

MISSED MENSES/AMENORRHEA

Women may present with a chief complaint of amenorrhea, or missed menses. Primary amenorrhea is defined as the lack of menarche by age 13 in a young woman without breast development, or 15 in a woman with breast development. True secondary amenorrhea is defined as the unintentional absence of menses for 6 consecutive months in a patient with a history of irregular menses, and unintentional absence of menses in a patient for 3 months with a history of regular menses. Most women will present with a missed menses. It is important to make this differentiation because many women will experience one missed menses, but will spontaneously bleed within the next 4 to 6 weeks. Once you have determined whether the patient is experiencing a missed menses, primary amenorrhea, or secondary amenorrhea, you can begin to formulate your differential diagnosis.[1]

All women who present with a missed menses must be ruled out for pregnancy. The urine human chorionic gonadotropin (HCG) may be positive when the serum beta-HCG reaches 20 to 25 IU/mL. The serum beta-HCG may be positive when the beta-HCG reaches 10 IU/mL. The negative predictive value for a urine beta-HCG is 98% and it is 95% sensitive.[1] Therefore, a urine HCG is an acceptable screening test to rule out pregnancy.

Differential Diagnosis

The differential diagnosis must be separated into primary and secondary amenorrhea. Primary amenorrhea may be due to chromosomal anomalies that produce a hypogonadic state (Kallman syndrome and Turner syndrome) or structural anomalies, such as imperforate hymen or cervical/Müellerian agenesis or dysgenesis.

- Primary without breast development:
  - Hypogonadic (Kallman syndrome, Turner syndrome)
  - 17-hydroxylase deficiency
- Primary with breast development and abnormal Müellerian structures:
  - Chromosomal abnormalities
  - Cervical and/or Müellerian agenesis or dysgenesis
- Secondary:
  - Pregnancy
  - Asherman's syndrome
  - Pituitary dysfunction
  - Hyperandrogenism
  - Prolactinemia
  - Premature ovarian failure
  - Hypothyroidism
  - Anorexia nervosa
  - Poor nutrition, extreme stress, extreme exercise

History

The HPI needs to focus on precisely how long the patient has been experiencing symptoms and rule in and out the etiologies on your differential diagnosis. Primary amenorrhea will usually require karyotype testing as over half of patients will have a chromosomal or structural abnormality. Thus, the following history will focus on the patient who presents with secondary amenorrhea, a more commonly encountered chief complaint.

- Onset, duration, and timing:
  ○ What is the patient's gravida and para status?
  ○ At what age was menarche? Was it spontaneous?
  ○ Did the patient have previously normal menses before this episode of amenorrhea?
  ○ Has this ever happened before? If so, what worked to help the patient experience a menses?
  ○ Has the patient had any uterine instrumentation (Asherman's syndrome)?
  ○ Has the patient been experiencing weight gain, skin changes, or changes in appetite or energy level (hypothyroidism, pregnancy, polycystic ovarian syndrome [PCOS])?
  ○ Is the patient taking any medications (hyperprolactinemia from medications)?
  ○ Recent intentional weight loss (anorexia)?
  ○ Is the patient exercising excessively?
  ○ Any vision changes/diplopia (prolactinoma)?
  ○ Milky nipple discharge (galactorrhea)?
  ○ History of infertility?
  ○ Currently trying to conceive?
  ○ Any contraception being used currently? Progestin-based contraception commonly causes secondary amenorrhea with continued use, and a change in oral contraception can cause secondary amenorrhea as well.

CLINICAL PEARL: A patient with signs of hyperandrogenism should be tested for PCOS. The presence of multiple follicular cysts on the ovaries is not essential for the diagnosis. Patients with PCOS tend to be hirsute, have abdominal adiposity, insulin resistance, and low level of sex hormone binding globulin (SHBG).

  ○ Associated symptoms: Think about the nongynecologic causes of secondary amenorrhea and continue to ask questions that may help you further narrow your differential diagnosis. This may be an appropriate time to ask the patient whether she is seeking to conceive or would like to prevent conception.

> **CLINICAL PEARL:** Sometimes patients will tell you that that they have not had a menses in months, but upon further questioning, they may admit to spotting or light bleeding (oligomenorrhea).

Past Medical History Specific to Complaint

- Endocrine: Thyroid disease, diabetes mellitus, known pituitary disorders, and PCOS.
- GI: Celiac disease or GI motility disorders.
- Renal: Chronic renal disease.
- Cardiovascular: History of (or current diagnosis of) hypertension.
- Psychiatric: History of psychiatric disorders.
- Trauma: History of head trauma.

Past Surgical History

- Ask about a history of uterine instrumentation (dilation and curettage, elective abortions, and hysteroscopic myomectomy).

Medications

- Thoroughly review the patient's medication list because many antipsychotic and antidepressant medications can cause hyperprolactinemia.
- Metoclopramide is used for GI motility disorders and nausea and can cause hyperprolactinemia.
- Verapamil and methyldopa can affect prolactin and thus can cause secondary amenorrhea.

Social History

- Heavy marijuana and opioid use have been implicated in hyperprolactinemia.
- Ask about social support networks if you suspect anorexia nervosa.

Physical Examination

Your physical examination needs to be a bit more comprehensive when evaluating a patient with amenorrhea because you have to think systematically. There can be physical clues to a diagnosis that, unless you looked, you would miss. See Table 1.5 for common physical examination findings and their associated clinical conditions, and Table 1.6 for common abnormal physical examination and laboratory findings that support or confirm the diagnosis of each condition listed.

TABLE 1.5 Correlating Physical Exam Findings With Pathologic Conditions

Body or Organ System	Physical Exam Finding	Associated Clinical Condition
General appearance	Webbed neck, short stature	Turner syndrome
	Hirsutism	PCOS
Vital signs	Hypertension	17-hydroxylase deficiency
	Hypotension	Anorexia nervosa, hypothyroidism
	BMI <17.5	Anorexia nervosa
HEENT	Anosmia	Kallman syndrome
	Bitemporal hemianopsia	Pituitary adenoma
Thyroid	Goiter, nodularity	Thyroid dysfunction
Breasts	Galactorrhea	Pituitary adenoma, medication side effect, pregnancy
Abdomen	Striae	Cushing syndrome
	Central adiposity	PCOS
Vulva and perineum	Absent vulva	Chromosomal abnormalities
Vagina	Vaginal dimple	Chromosomal abnormalities
	Bulge at introitus	Imperforate hymen, hematocolpos
	Decreased rugae, pale epithelium	Premature ovarian failure
Cervix	Bluish-purple discoloration	Chadwick's sign (pregnancy)
	Absent cervix	Müellerian agenesis
Adnexa	Enlarged adnexa	PCOS
Bimanual Exam	Absent uterus	Müellerian agenesis

BMI, body mass index; HEENT, head, ears, eyes, nose, throat; PCOS, polycystic ovarian syndrome.

TABLE 1.6 Correlating Pathologic Conditions With Objective Findings

Clinical Condition	Notable Physical Exam Findings	Notable Laboratory Findings
Turner syndrome	Short stature, webbed neck	45,X most common
17-hydroxylase deficiency	Absent secondary sexual characteristics	Hypertension and hypokalemia; 46,XX
Müellerian agenesis/ dysgenesis	Ambiguous genitalia; primary amenorrhea	46,XY
Primary ovarian insufficiency/premature ovarian failure	Secondary amenorrhea, menopause before age 40 years, vasomotor symptoms	May have elevated inhibin B, elevated FSH, low estradiol

(continued)

TABLE 1.6 Correlating Pathologic Conditions With Objective Findings (*continued*)

Clinical Condition	Notable Physical Exam Findings	Notable Laboratory Findings
Hyperprolactinemia[a]	Variable, depending on underlying etiology	Elevated prolactin
Congenital adrenal hyperplasia[b]	Atypical genitalia	Extremely elevated 17-hydroxyprogesterone
Polycystic ovarian syndrome	Hirsutism, acne, virilization of genitalia, central adiposity	Insulin resistance, elevated androgens, low sex hormone binding globulin (SHBG)

[a] Always ask about a patient's medications. Certain drugs are more likely to cause an elevated prolactin, including metoclopramide and some antipsychotics.
[b] Newborns are screened for congenital adrenal hyperplasia (CAH) at birth in the United States. Newborns can have a salt wasting adrenal crisis.

Diagnostic Plan

The diagnostic workup of a patient with amenorrhea depends upon whether the patient has primary or secondary amenorrhea and whether the HCG is negative.

- HCG (urine qualitative or serum quantitative beta-HCG)
  - Evaluate to rule out pregnancy, the most common cause of secondary amenorrhea.
- Thyroid-stimulating hormone (TSH): A serum test for thyroid function
  - Evaluate for hypo- or hyperthyroidism; a normal TSH with an elevated prolactin indicates a microadenoma or prolactinoma.
- Prolactin: A measurement of serum prolactin
  - Evaluate for hyperprolactinemia. A normal prolactin rules out hyperprolactinemia.
- Progestin challenge used if the HCG is negative and the TSH and prolactin are normal
  - Evaluate for the presence or absence of a progestin-withdrawal bleed that could help diagnose anovulation.
- Estrogen+progestin challenge is used if a patient does not have a withdrawal bleed from a progestin challenge
  - Evaluate for an outflow problem if no bleeding occurs; if bleeding occurs, the follicle-stimulating hormone (FSH) and luteinizing hormone (LH) should be checked next.
- FSH: It is best to check on day 3 in a menstruating woman
  - Evaluate for low FSH (and LH) in the presence of a withdrawal bleed, which indicates hypogonadic hypogonadism.
  - Evaluate for elevated FSH (and LH) in the presence of a withdrawal bleed, which indicates ovarian failure.

- LH: See FSH
- SHBG
  - Evaluate for PCOS. A low SHBG indicates PCOS.
- Karyotype testing is reserved for patients with primary amenorrhea and in whom you suspect a chromosomal abnormality

Initial Management

- The management of a patient with secondary amenorrhea largely depends on the underlying pathology, if present.
- If the HCG is negative and the TSH and prolactin are normal, patients should undergo a progestin-withdrawal challenge.
  - Medroxyprogesterone acetate 10 mg each day for 10 days is prescribed to the patient.
  - Within 2 weeks, the patient should have a withdrawal bleed.
  - The presence of a withdrawal bleed indicates adequate endometrial estrogen exposure.
  - If a patient does not experience a withdrawal bleed, this could indicate inadequate estrogen exposure or an outflow problem.
  - It is important to confirm that the patient both picked up the prescription for the progestin and took it as directed.
- A prolonged hypoestrogenic state can result in reduced bone mineral density.
  - Consider ordering bone mineral density testing and appropriate measures implemented to rebuild bone, including lifestyle and possible pharmacologic interventions per current guidelines.
- Chronic anovulation is a risk factor for endometrial hyperplasia.
  - A combination hormonal contraceptive often allows the patient to experience withdrawal bleeding each month, while also protecting against unwanted pregnancy.
  - Other options include daily or cyclic progestins or a progestin-secreting IUS.
- Women with PCOS who do not wish to conceive should have adequate counseling on the need for contraception because spontaneous ovulation can occur.

Key Points . . .

- Patients with primary amenorrhea must be evaluated for karyotype abnormalities that could cause anatomic anomalies and the presence or absence of imperforate hymen leading to hematocolpos.
- Patients with amenorrhea should be ruled out for pregnancy.
- Patients with chronic anovulation and amenorrhea must be provided with a progestin to protect against endometrial hyperplasia.
- Once pregnancy or other systemic disease has been ruled out, patients should undergo a progestin -withdrawal challenge, unless contraindications exist for use of progestin.

REFERENCE

1. Simon A, Chang WY, DeCherny AH. Amenorrhea. In: DeCherney A, DeCherney AH, Nathan L, Laufer N, Roman AS, et al, ed. *Current Diagnosis and Treatment Obstetrics and Gynecology*. New York, NY: McGraw-Hill Medical; 2013:889–899.

PELVIC PAIN

The differential diagnosis for pelvic pain can be long and overwhelming, so it is helpful to categorize the pain as either acute, cyclic, or chronic. See Tables 1.7 and 1.8 for the differential diagnosis of acute and chronic pelvic pain. As previously stated, you must also assess whether the patient is of reproductive age or menopausal. Always ask when the LMP occurred, whether the patient has had any pelvic surgical procedures, and whether the patient has ever experienced this type of pain prior to the visit. As a rule, all patients of reproductive age who still have a uterus and at least one ovary are pregnant until proven otherwise.[1,2]

Painful menses, or dysmenorrhea, is the most commonly encountered cause of pelvic pain.[1] Dysmenorrhea can be further classified as primary or secondary. Primary dysmenorrhea generally occurs within the first few years after menarche and is due to prostaglandin production. As such, it is generally responsive to nonsteroidal anti-inflammatory medications (NSAIDs). Secondary dysmenorrhea is generally caused by an underlying pathology, including endometriosis, adenomyosis, and ovarian cysts. Often, secondary dysmenorrhea is amenable to NSAIDs as well, but addressing the underlying pathology is important.

It is important to remember that pelvic pain is a symptom, so a careful history and physical examination can often help you diagnose the underlying etiology and provide appropriate treatment.

Differential Diagnosis

TABLE 1.7 Differential Diagnosis of Acute Pelvic Pain in a Menstruating Woman

Gynecologic	Nongynecologic
Ectopic pregnancy	Appendicitis
Ruptured ovarian cyst	Exacerbation of inflammatory bowel disease
Ovarian torsion	Diverticulitis

(continued)

TABLE 1.7 Differential Diagnosis of Acute Pelvic Pain in a Menstruating Woman (*continued*)

Gynecologic	Nongynecologic
Pelvic inflammatory disease	Severe constipation
Tubo-ovarian abscess	Nephrolithiasis
Endometritis	Urinary tract infection
IUS perforation	Pelvic vein thrombosis
Other trauma	

IUS, intrauterine system.

TABLE 1.8 Differential Diagnosis of Chronic Pelvic Pain in a Menstruating Woman

Gynecologic	Nongynecologic
Primary or secondary dysmenorrhea	Interstitial cystitis
Ovarian cysts	Irritable bowel syndrome
Endometriosis	Inflammatory bowel disease
Leiomyomata	Gastrointestinal neoplasms
Adenomyosis	Psychological issue
Pelvic congestion	Fibromyalgia
Ovarian neoplasms	
Pelvic adhesions	

History

The gynecologic history must always include the patient's gravida and para status, LMP, and, if of reproductive age and sexually active with men, what the patient is using for contraception or has used in the past.

- Onset, duration, and timing: Ask the patient about when the pain started, how often it occurs, and how long it lasts. Pain that occurred one time after intercourse that only lasted a few minutes is less likely to be endometriosis. Chronic pelvic pain is pain that has been present for at least 6 months and negatively effects a patient's quality of life.[1] If pain occurs with intercourse, you must differentiate between deep dyspareunia, pain with intromission (insertion), or midvaginal pain. Pelvic pain that occurs within a few weeks of a pelvic procedure or childbirth can be endometritis, and pelvic pain after an intrauterine system (IUS) has been inserted can indicate a perforation.

> **CLINICAL PEARL:** Acute onset of pelvic pain in a menstruating woman is an ectopic pregnancy until proven otherwise. Ovarian torsion should be ruled out as well.

- Provoking/alleviating factors: Have the patient describe what makes the pain better, if anything, and what either causes pain or makes the pain worse. Primary dysmenorrhea is often alleviated with NSAIDS.

> **CLINICAL PEARL:** Painful intercourse (dyspareunia) is often a hallmark of endometriosis, but can also occur in patients with ovarian cysts, pelvic inflammatory disease (PID), adenomyosis, and a history of sexual abuse. The most common cause of dyspareunia in postmenopausal women is vulvovaginal atrophy.

- Quality: It is helpful to have the patient describe what she is feeling in greater detail. For example, some patients describe the pain of large leiomyomas as a dull ache with a sensation of pelvic "fullness" due to its compression on pelvic nerves.

> **CLINICAL PEARL:** Chronic pelvic pain is usually described as achy and dull, whereas acute pelvic pain is usually described as sharp.

- Radiation/Location: Ask the patient to try and locate where the pain is occurring. Does it feel as if it is deep in the pelvis or vagina? Does the pain radiate to any other areas? Many women have a poor understanding of their genital anatomy, so it is important to help assess where the pain is occurring.

> **CLINICAL PEARL:** Pelvic or abdominal pain is present in almost all patients with an ectopic pregnancy.

- Severity: You can ask the patient to grade her pain on a scale of 0 to 10, but sometimes it helps to ask the patient to describe how the pain interferes with her daily routine.

> **CLINICAL PEARL:** When patients describe their pain as acute and severe, ovarian torsion and ectopic pregnancy must be in your differential diagnosis and quickly ruled out.

- Associated symptoms: The presence or absence of nausea, vomiting, diaphoresis, and apprehension must be assessed. Pain that produces these autonomic symptoms can indicate an etiology that carries an increased risk of morbidity and mortality, such as an ectopic pregnancy. Ask the patient about whether there is any association with vaginal bleeding, urination, defecation, or intercourse.

> **CLINICAL PEARL:** A patient with chronic pelvic pain and dyspareunia who has had a negative pelvic ultrasound and diagnostic laparoscopy should be assessed for interstitial cystitis.

Past Medical History and Review of Symptoms Specific to Complaint

- OB/GYN: Always obtain the patient's gravida and para status, with careful attention to whether the patient had been diagnosed with an ectopic pregnancy in the past. Assess whether the patient has ever been diagnosed with ovarian cysts or pelvic inflammatory disease (PID), or whether the patient has an IUS.

> **CLINICAL PEARL:** A risk factor for ectopic pregnancy is a history of an ectopic pregnancy.

- Urinary: Ask about dysuria, hematuria, frequency, urgency, incontinence, and difficulty emptying the bladder.

> **CLINICAL PEARL:** Interstitial cystitis can present with chronic urinary tract infections (UTIs) and dysuria with negative urine cultures. However, gross hematuria is rare. Patients with nephrolithiasis will always have hematuria.

- Gastrointestinal (GI): Ask whether the patient has constipation or diarrhea; abdominal pain; dyspepsia; bleeding with bowel movements; changes with bowel movements, including frequency, shape, and color of stool; changes in appetite; and nausea and vomiting. Frequency of urination can be due to a mass effect. Constipation or difficulty with defecation could be caused by a mass or pelvic organ prolapse.

> **CLINICAL PEARL:** Early satiety is a common finding in women with advanced ovarian cancer.

- Musculoskeletal: Chronic pain in multiple areas of the body could indicated fibromyalgia.

> **CLINICAL PEARL:** Chronic pelvic pain in a patient without observable pathology may be pelvic myofascial pain. Referral to a physical therapist who specializes in pelvic floor dysfunction may be helpful.

- Hematologic: Ask the patient about a history of blood dyscrasias and whether she has had a recent episode of prolonged immobilization, such as a long car drive or plane ride.

CLINICAL PEARL: Assessing the patient for hypercoagulable risk factors is important because a pelvic venous thrombosis, although rare, can present as pelvic pain.

- Psychological: Ask about the patient's psychological history, including any anxiety, depressive disorders, and history of sexual abuse.

CLINICAL PEARL: Always ask the patient about sexual practices and whether she is satisfied with her current partner(s). It can be a good way to begin a conversation about intimate partner violence and sexual health.

Social History

- Safety: Does the patient feel safe in her home and in her relationship? You may discover domestic abuse, sexual abuse, or human trafficking in a patient with chronic pelvic pain.

CLINICAL PEARL: Know which agency is available for referrals regarding domestic abuse and human trafficking.

- Tobacco, alcohol, illicit drugs: Tobacco smoke is a risk factor for a multitude of pathologies, including ectopic pregnancy.

CLINICAL PEARL: A patient who engages in high-risk sexual behaviors is at risk for developing PID and other sexually transmitted infections, including HIV.

Physical Examination

A focused physical examination aimed at further narrowing the differential diagnosis is the essential next step in evaluating a patient. Specific physical examination findings can help support, confirm, or rule out various diagnoses. Table 1.9 will help you correlate physical exam findings with various pathologies.

TABLE 1.9 Correlating Physical Exam Findings With Pathologic Conditions

Body or Organ System	Physical Exam Finding	Associated Clinical Condition
General appearance	Diaphoretic, anxious	Ectopic pregnancy, ovarian torsion, ruptured hemorrhagic ovarian cyst
Vital signs	Tachycardia, hypotension	Ruptured ectopic pregnancy, ruptured hemorrhagic ovarian cyst
	Fever	PID, endometritis, pelvic abscess
Abdomen	Tenderness on palpation	PID, endometritis, pelvic abscess, ruptured ovarian cyst
	Ascites	Ovarian cancer
Vulva and perineum	Tears, ecchymosis, abrasions	Trauma
Vagina	Blood	Trauma, menstruation
Cervix	Os open, dilated	Spontaneous abortion
	Cervical purulence	Sexually transmitted infections, cervicitis
Adnexa	Mass	Ovarian cyst, ovarian cancer (ectopic pregnancies will rarely be palpable on bimanual)
Bimanual exam	Cervical motion tenderness	PID, cervicitis
	Nodules along uterosacral ligaments	Endometriosis
	Tenderness or nodules in the pouch of Douglas	Endometriosis, malignancy, PID
	Enlarged uterus	Leiomyoma, pregnancy, adenomyosis

PID, pelvic inflammatory disease.

Diagnostic Plan

- Beta-HCG: All patients who are of reproductive age who still have a uterus should have a pregnancy test. A urine qualitative pregnancy test is sufficient in most patients with pelvic pain. If the pregnancy test is positive, the patient should have a quantitative beta-HCG as well so that clinical correlations can be made.
  - Evaluate for: Any disorder related to pregnancy and to rule out pregnancy-related pathologies. A positive test warrants further workup, and a negative test means that you can cross off pregnancy-related problems in your differential.
    - A positive quantitative beta-HCG should double by 72 hours after the initial draw in a normal pregnancy.
    - Patients with a serum beta-HCG >2,000 IU/mL with no gestational sac on ultrasound are considered to have an ectopic pregnancy until proven otherwise.
- Serum progesterone: Can help to differentiate a normal intrauterine pregnancy (IUP) from an abnormal pregnancy.
  - Evaluate for a normal IUP.

- Patients with a serum progesterone greater than 20 ng/mL are much more likely to have normal IUPs. Patients with an ectopic usually have serum progesterone less than 5 ng/mL and always less than 20 ng/mL.
- Urine dipstick: This is an inexpensive test used to screen for cystitis, hematuria, ketonuria, and glucosuria.
  - Evaluate for cystitis (UTI). Nitrites, leukocyte esterase, and blood have limited sensitivity and specificity. If the clinical suspicion is high for cystitis, particularly in pregnancy, urine microscopy and culture should be ordered, but empiric treatment can be considered if the symptoms are consistent with a UTI.
    - If a woman is menstruating, even with the slightest bit of spotting, the dipstick can show positive for blood. Other reasons why blood may be evident on urine dipstick include dehydration and exercise. Leukocyte esterase and nitrite can occur with contamination of either the specimen or the dipstick itself.
- Sexually transmitted infection (STI) testing: This may be necessary in a patient with pelvic pain, cervicitis, vaginal discharge, and who is at risk for STIs.
  - Generally speaking, acute trichomonas, bacterial vaginosis, and vaginal candidiasis do not cause pelvic pain. The Centers for Disease Control and Prevention (CDC) maintains that there is no single reliable screening test for PID but that the absence of white blood cells on wet prep could effectively rule out PID as long as other clinical criteria have not been met. See Chapter 2, Common Disease Entities in Gynecology, for a more thorough discussion of PID diagnosis and treatment.
- Pelvic ultrasound: This is an excellent way to image the pelvic organs when structural issues and pregnancy are suspected.
  - Evaluate for ovarian masses, leiomyomata, pregnancy (location: intrauterine, ectopic; viability: fetal cardiac activity, molar).
    - Often, PA students and new PAs may have a difficult time differentiating adnexal masses and uterine masses, such as leiomyoma, on bimanual examination.
- Diagnostic laparoscopy: A surgical procedure that can be done if ultrasonography and other noninvasive testing have not revealed a pathology.
  - Evaluate for endometriosis, adhesions, masses, and pelvic inflammatory disease.
    - All laparoscopies are diagnostic in that you never know what you will encounter when you enter the pelvis.
- Cystoscopy: Visualization of the bladder. Some OB/GYNs perform this procedure in the office. You may have to refer to a urogynecologist if your practice does not have a cystoscope.
  - Evaluate for interstitial cystitis, bladder neoplasia.

- Colonoscopy: To be considered when you suspect gastrointestinal pathology.
  - Evaluate for polyps, neoplasia, diverticulitis/diverticulosis.

> **CLINICAL PEARL:** Transvaginal ultrasonography is superior to transabdominal imaging when evaluating the adnexa, cervix, cul-de-sac, and the endometrium. It is also the preferred method of imaging during the first trimester of pregnancy.

Initial Management

- If the patient is found to be pregnant, determine whether the pregnancy is viable. For more information about the management of first-trimester pregnancy complications, see Chapter 3, Common Disease Entities in Obstetrics.
- Patients with chronic pelvic pain should have an ultrasound and diagnostic laparoscopy to rule out pathology that cannot be diagnosed with noninvasive testing.
- Opioids are never indicated for the treatment of chronic pelvic pain and should be used judiciously in acute pelvic pain.
- NSAIDs are the mainstay of pharmacologic treatment of pelvic pain, particularly dysmenorrhea.
- Hormonal therapies are effective for endometriosis and secondary dysmenorrhea without underlying pathology. Be careful to screen for contraindications.
- If an infectious etiology is suspected, treat according to the most current CDC guidelines.
- Consider referral to a women's health physical therapist once life-threatening etiologies have been ruled out.

Key Points . . .

- Pelvic pain must be differentiated between acute and chronic.
- Women of reproductive age should be ruled out for pregnancy unless they have had a hysterectomy or premature ovarian failure.
- A careful history will allow you the opportunity to stratify the patient into risk categories. High-risk etiologies of acute pelvic pain in a menstruating woman include ectopic pregnancy and ovarian torsion.
- Think about the pelvic and abdominal anatomy. What organs are located where, and what could be causing pain in those areas?
- Be sure to ask about urinary and abdominal symptoms as the presence of absence of symptoms can help refine the differential.

REFERENCES

1. Hacker N, Gambone J, Hobel C, eds. *Hacker & Moore's Essentials of Obstetrics and Gynecology.* 6th ed. Philadelphia, PA: Elsevier; 2016.
2. DeCherney AH, Roman AS, Nathan L, et al., eds. *Current Diagnosis and Treatment: Obstetrics and Gynecology.* 11th ed. New York, NY: McGraw-Hill Medical; 2013.

Prenatal Visit

Women have regularly scheduled visits for prenatal checks, but will sometimes make an appointment for other complaints. This section reviews what should occur at a regularly scheduled prenatal visit. For more information on commonly encountered problems in pregnancy, see Chapter 3, Common Disease Entities in Obstetrics.[1-3]

Every visit is an opportunity to provide patient education and counseling, and to screen for any new issues. You should also review all labs and imaging to ensure the medical record is complete.

ACOG recommends the following schedule for prenatal visits in a gravid patient without any comorbid issues or complications: a prenatal visit every 4 weeks until 28 weeks, every 2 weeks until 36 weeks, and weekly until delivery.

It is recommended that each gravid patient receive laboratory and STI testing at her first visit. These tests include a CBC, blood type, antibody screen, rubella titer, hepatitis (hepatitis B surface antigen [HBsAg]), HIV, urine dipstick and culture, syphilis (Venereal Disease Research Laboratory [VDRL]/rapid plasma reagin [RPR]), chlamydia, and gonorrhea, as outlined in Table 1.10

All women should be offered genetic testing as appropriate, per their risk assessments. Women at high risk of tuberculosis (TB) should be screened for TB. Women with a history of diabetes or who have other risk factors for diabetes may be assessed with a hemoglobin A1c (HbA1c) or 1-hour oral glucose challenge test as well.

The first prenatal visit also includes a comprehensive review of the patient's past medical history, including gravida and para history, genetics history, social history, and physical examination. It is also an important time to assess the patient's risk for medical and social problems during pregnancy and postpartum.

Some professional societies consider a woman to be of advanced maternal age (AMA) if she conceived at 35 years of age or older, whereas others consider AMA if she is 35 years or older at delivery. Women who are AMA are at risk of carrying a fetus with chromosomal abnormalities, intrauterine fetal demise, and other obstetric complications. Risk is proportional to the patient's age. Risk increases if the patient is a tobacco user and/or is obese. Patients who are AMA should be referred to a maternal–fetal medicine specialist for genetic screening and possible chorionic villus sampling, amniocentesis, and other ancillary testing as necessary.

A detailed obstetric history will include information about all prior deliveries. You must document the date of the delivery, the gestational age of the fetus, length of labor, birth weight, type of delivery (vaginal delivery or cesarean), place of delivery, breastfeeding duration and whether the patient required a lactation consultant, and a narrative of any complications.

Examples of complications that need to be documented include precipitous delivery (duration of first and second stages of labor less than 2 hours with rapid delivery of the fetus); an infant positive for Group B *Streptococcus*; infant who was placed for adoption; if infant had any congenital issues; postpartum hemorrhage; placenta previa or accreta; amnionitis; anesthesia complications; perineal tears; forceps delivery; and vacuum-assisted delivery.

The patient's past medical history has specific questions that must be asked. These include the following:

- Drug or latex allergies
- Food allergies
- Neurological disease (such as a seizure disorder)
- History of breast surgery or disease
- Asthma or TB
- Heart disease
- Hypertension
- Cancer of any kind
- Hematologic disorders, such as thalassemia, sickle cell carrier, thrombocytopenia, Protein C deficiency
- Anemia
- Gastrointestinal disorders such as Crohn's disease, ulcerative colitis
- Hepatic disease, including hepatitis and history of cholestatic disease
- Renal disease, including urinary tract infections, nephrolithiasis
- Venous thromboembolic events
- Diabetes, including type 1, type 2, and gestational diabetes
- Autoimmune disorders
- Dermatologic disorders
- Surgical history, including any vaginal/obstetrical surgeries with date and reason, if known
- Anesthetic complications that may not have been uncovered as described previously
- History of blood transfusions, including date and reason, if known

- History of infertility, including use of assisted reproductive technologies, including in vitro fertilization
- Polycystic ovarian syndrome
- History of cervical dysplasia
- STIs
- Psychiatric disorders
- Postpartum depression, perinatal depression, major depression

  The social history must include the following questions:

- Use of illicit drugs, opioids, alcohol, and tobacco
  ○ Ask about vaping as well
- Interpersonal violence
- History of trauma

Genetic screening is important in all patients and is done at the initial visit. It is important to ask whether the disease has occurred in the patient, the father of the baby, or any other family member. Although cystic fibrosis screening is a part of the initial obstetric screening panel, a patient with a family history of any of the other diseases listed here (and others not specifically listed, such as Huntington's disease), should be referred for genetic counseling. Most maternal–fetal medicine specialists will have a geneticist on staff.

Specific diseases that must be assessed include the following:

- Congenital heart defects
- Neural tube defects
- Hemoglobinopathies
- Hemophilia
- Cystic fibrosis
- Chromosomal abnormalities
- Tay-Sachs disease
- Intellectual disabilities
- Autism
- Recurrent pregnancy loss
- Stillbirth
- Phenylketonuria (PKU)
- Muscular dystrophy
- Any other genetic disorders not listed earlier

It is also important to evaluate potential teratogen exposure. At this first visit, you must ask the patient about possible exposures that could negatively affect the patient and/or the pregnancy. If the patient has an exposure, consider referral to a maternal–fetal medicine specialist.

- Use of prescription medications
  ○ If the patient is on any prescription medication, use a reliable drug-reference guide to make sure it is considered safe in pregnancy.

- ○ Although the Food and Drug Administration (FDA) recently changed the pregnancy and lactation drug labeling from A, B, C, D, and X to a narrative describing possible or known adverse effects, some drugs are well known to cause birth defects.
- ○ Medications known to cause birth defects include certain antiseizure medications such as phenytoin, valproic acid, carbamazepine, lamotrigine, isotretinoin, misoprostol, lithium, statins, alcohol, androgens, tetracycline, warfarin, and methotrexate and other antineoplastic drugs.
- Use of over-the-counter medications
  - ○ NSAIDs should never be used in the third trimester as they can cause premature closure of the ductus arteriosus of the fetus.[4]
  - ○ There is an association with NSAID use in the first trimester and early pregnancy loss.
- Excessive vitamin A
- Alcohol
- Illicit drugs
- Maternal diabetes
- Ionizing radiation

In addition, the patient's infectious disease history and risk are assessed. Questions that must be asked include the following:

- Any rash since last menstrual period
- Personal history of genital herpes
- Partner with genital herpes
- Known exposure to TB or live with someone who has TB
- Prior Group B *Streptococcus*-positive infant
- Known history of gonorrhea, chlamydia, HPV, PID, and syphilis
- HIV status, if known
- History of hepatitis
- Travel outside of the United States by the patient or partner
- Possible exposure to Zika virus (should be assessed at each trimester)
- Any other pertinent information

The patient's immunization history must be documented.

- Tdap: Patients should receive Tdap during each pregnancy within 27 to 36 weeks' gestation
- Influenza: Nasal influenza vaccine should not be used
- Measles, mumps, and rubella (MMR)
- Hepatitis A if indicated
- Hepatitis B
- Meningococcal vaccine
- Pneumococcal vaccine

The intial obstetric physical exam is a complete physical exam. Document the patient's prepregnancy weight, if known. Measuring the patient's current weight and height and calculating her body mass index (BMI) are important to assess for possible complications of pregnancy and delivery. Other elements of the physical exam that must be completed are the following:

- HEENT
- Dentition
- Thyroid
- Breasts
- Lungs
- Heart
- Abdomen
- Extremities (note any range of motion [ROM] limitations)
- Skin
- Lymph nodes
- Vulva
- Vagina
- Cervix
- Uterine size
- Adnexa
- Rectum
- Pelvimetry
    - If a patient has had a prior vaginal delivery, you can document this section by writing "Patient had prior normal spontaneous vaginal delivery (NSVD)." Some providers write, "Proven pelvis."

The estimated date of delivery (EDD) is an important component of the initial exam. If the patient's LMP is known, you can calculate the EDD with the LMP using a gestation wheel or the electronic medical record will perform the calculation for you. If on the initial exam there is a discrepancy, such as a uterus that is smaller or larger than estimated gestational weeks by EDD, the finding must be documented and followed up with ultrasound. Remember that if the patient is sure about her LMP and the ultrasound is within 2 weeks of the EDD by LMP, you can use the LMP date. Ultrasounds for dating pregnancy are really only useful in the first trimester and still have a 2-week margin of error. If the patient underwent in vitro fertilization, document the date of the transfer.

Subsequent prenatal visits must include documentation of the following:

- Gestational age by weeks
- Patient's weight
- Blood pressure
- Urine for protein and glucose (and if symptomatic, check for blood, leukocyte esterase, and nitrites; if positive, send urine for culture)
- Presence of fetal movement (after the first trimester)
- Preterm labor signs (third trimester) or symptoms

- Fetal heart rate
- Fundal height
- Fetal presentation (at 36 weeks or sooner if the patient is in preterm labor)
- Edema
- Cervical exam (at 36 weeks or sooner if the patient is symptomatic): dilation, effacement, station; length by ultrasound if indicated
- Recent travel outside of the United States
- Next appointment in weeks
- Your initials
- Any other comments that are necessary, including any changes in health status, social situation, and so on. It is also helpful to document when the patient has registered at whichever hospital she has chosen for delivery. Typically, patients register between 34 and 38 weeks.

  Important points to remember:

- Fetal heart tones (FHTs) with a Doppler can be heard by 12 to 14 weeks, depending on the adiposity of the patient.
- The fetal heart rate can vary between 120 and 170 beats per minute, sometimes more than twice the rate of the gravid patient.
- Some women can feel fetal movements as early as 16 weeks, but some women, particularly primigravidas, may not feel fetal movements until 24 weeks. This first sensation of fetal movement is called *quickening*.
- After 26 to 28 weeks, gravid patients should regularly feel fetal movements, or kicks.
  - A decrease in movement calls for further testing with a nonstress test (NST) and possibly a biophysical profile (BPP.)
- ACOG recommends that pregnant patients should be aware of fetal movements.
  - Documentation regarding patient education of fetal kick counts should occur.
- At each prenatal visit, women should have their blood pressure and weight checked, a urine test for protein and glucose, and after 12 weeks, a check of FHTs.
- Starting at 28 weeks, patients should be asked about fetal movements and preterm labor symptoms.
- Each visit is an opportunity to provide patient education, counseling, and anticipatory guidance.
  - During the first trimester, ask about the possibility of the patient requiring a Women, Infants, and Children (WIC) form.
  - During the third trimester, ask about availability of approved car seats, social support networks, plans for lactation consultation, postpartum contraception, risk for postpartum depression, and plans to return to work when appropriate.
- For a comprehensive review of patient education talking points in pregnancy, please see Chapter 5, Patient Education and Counseling in OB/GYN.

Diagnostic Plan

Once you have established a viable intrauterine pregnancy, follow ACOG recommendations regarding when to use diagnostics. Table 1.10 provides an outline of the most commonly used tests during pregnancy.

Ultrasound in the first trimester:

- Gestational sac (GS): Not useful for dating a pregnancy; an empty GS larger than 25 mm could indicate an anembryonic pregnancy
  - Expectant management with follow-up ultrasound in 10 days to 2 weeks and correlation with beta-HCG.
- Yolk sac (YS): Visualized by 5 weeks' gestation
- Crown–rump length (CRL): Accuracy of gestational age within 5 to 7 days up to 14 weeks' gestation
- Cardiac activity: Should be seen at 5.5 to 6 weeks' gestation
- A first-trimester ultrasound (<13w6d) is the most accurate way of dating a pregnancy when the LMP is in question
  - Prior to 8w6d, if the EDD by CRL is more than 5-days different than the LMP, a follow-up ultrasound is justified in 10 days to 2 weeks
  - Between 9 weeks and 13w6d, if the EDD by CRL is more than 7-days different, a follow-up ultrasound is justified
- Early first-trimester ultrasounds are useful to evaluate for possible ectopic and molar pregnancy, ensure a pregnancy is viable and in the uterus, screen for fetal aneuploidy and other early abnormalities such as anencephaly, to date a pregnancy, evaluate vaginal bleeding in early pregnancy, assess maternal pelvic masses, and determine the number of gestations in utero
- Confirming a viable intrauterine pregnancy (IUP) long before FHTs can be heard with a Doppler also improves patient satisfaction

Physical Examination

- Fundal height. All gravid patients at 20 weeks until about 36 weeks should have a fundal height measured and documented.
  - Measurement of fundal height is accomplished with a tape measure. Begin with one hand holding the tape measure at 0 cm at the upper edge of the pubic symphysis. Then measure the distance from that point to the top of the uterine fundus. The distance in centimeters should correlate with the gestational age, +/− 2 weeks, in a singleton pregnancy.
  - Think of this measurement as a way to track fetal growth. You want to see proportional growth over time.
  - Conditions that can cause a consistently higher (multiple gestation, polyhydramnios) or lower measurement (intrauterine growth restriction) are discussed in Chapter 3, Common Disease Entities in Obstetrics.
  - After about 36 weeks, the fetus may "drop" into the pelvis, thus the measurement becomes less accurate.

TABLE 1.10 Common Laboratory and Other Diagnostic Testing by Gestational Age

Gestational Age	Lab Testing	Other Diagnostics	Clinical Reason
First prenatal visit	CBC		Anemia
	Blood type and Rh		Blood type and Rh
	Antibody screen		Alloimmunization
	HBsAg		Hepatitis B immunity
	VDRL/RPR		Syphilis
	Rubella titer		Rubella immunity
	HIV		HIV
	Urine culture		Asymptomatic bacteriuria
	HbA1c or 1-hour oral glucose challenge test[b]		Gestational or preexisting diabetes
		Chlamydia and gonorrhea PCR	Chlamydia and gonorrhea infection
		Pelvic ultrasound	Viability, number of gestations, dating
		TB skin test	TB (if patient at risk)
10w0d and on	Cell-free DNA		Down syndrome
10–13w6d	PAPP-A and HCGa	Nuchal translucency	Down syndrome
		Chorionic villus sampling	Chromosomal abnormalities
15–20w0d		Amniocentesis	Fetal aneuplody Chromosomal abnormalities
	"Triple screen" HCG, AFP, uE3		Fetal aneuplody
	"Quad screen" HCG, AFP, uE3, inhibin A		Fetal aneuploidy
18–22 weeks		Ultrasound	Fetal survey
24–28 weeks	1-hour glucola		Gestational diabetes
	Hgb and HCT		Anemia
	Antibody screen		Alloimmunizaton
35–37 weeks	GBS		GBS colonization

[a]Often combined with quad screen, called *integrated screening*.
[b]May offer early screening for gestational diabetes mellitus (GDM) and diabetes mellitus (DM) if the patient has risk factors, but if early screen is negative, still need to do third trimester screen.
AFP, alpha-fetoprotein; CBC, complete blood count; GBS, group B *Streptococcus*; HbA1c, hemoglobin A1c; HBsAg, hepatitis B surface antigen; HCG, human chorionic gonadotropin; HCT, hematocrit; Hgb, hemoglobin; PAPP-A, pregnancy-associated plasma protein A; PCR, polymerase chain reaction; TB, tuberculosis; VDRL/RPR, Venereal Disease Research Laboratory/rapid plasma regain; uE3, unconjugated estriol.

- FHTs. As mentioned previously, FHTs can be heard with a hand held Doppler from about 12 to 14 weeks on. It is important to distinguish maternal pulse from FHTs. This can usually be easily accomplished by counting the beats. Normal FHTs can vary between 120 and 170 beats per minute.
  - ○ Sometimes it is difficult to hear FHTs in women with a protuberant, adipose abdomen, particularly during the early second trimester. If there is ever a question about FHTs, it is advisable to have your preceptor check. If they are still not audible, a limited ultrasound can be done to assess FHTs.
  - ○ Some women maintain that a "faster" heart rate is associated with a female fetus, whereas a "slower" heart rate is associated with a male fetus. This is simply untrue. The fetal heart rate will naturally fluctuate throughout the day, increasing during times when the fetus is active and decreasing during sleep cycles.
  - ○ Rarely, you may hear a fetal arrhythmia. If you have a concern about a true tachycardia or bradycardia, or an irregular rhythm, notify your preceptor immediately. The patient will need to have an ultrasound, an NST if clinically indicated, and will likely be referred to a maternal–fetal medicine specialist if an abnormality is detected.
- Pelvic examination. Generally speaking, a pelvic examination is done at the first prenatal visit and not again until 34 to 35 weeks, when the patient will have group B *Streptococcus* (GBS) testing.
  - ○ GBS testing involves taking a bacterial culture swab and performing a vagino–rectal swab. It is not necessary to check the patient's cervix at this time, but often a bimanual exam is performed to assess the presenting fetal part (head down [vertex/cephalic] or breech). However, a cervical check may reveal early dilation and effacement in an otherwise asymptomatic patient.
  - ○ Routine pelvic examinations during pregnancy are not necessary until the patient either complains of pelvic pain, cramping, contractions, or spotting. Some OB/GYNs will begin digital exams of the cervix at about 36 weeks to assess fetal presentation and cervical change. It is possible to palpate the presenting part during a digital exam but this requires experience.
  - ○ A digital exam should be avoided if a patient presents with bleeding in the third trimester until placenta previa has been ruled out with an ultrasound.
  - ○ If a patient presents with possible rupture of membranes, you must use sterile gloves and a sterile speculum to examine the patient prior to a digital exam.
- Cervix. Physical examination of the cervix during late pregnancy is a common source of frustration for students. Imagine having someone place an

object with which you are unfamiliar into a deep bowl of pudding that is placed in a paper bag. The person then asks you to close your eyes and (a) find the object and (b) measure the object in centimeters using only your two fingers.

○ When you are performing a digital exam on a pregnant patient in the third trimester, you will have to measure the width of the opening (dilation) of the cervical os in centimeters, and the amount of thinning (effacement), measured as a percentage.

○ Women who have had one or more deliveries often will walk around with a cervix that is dilated from 1 to 2 cm and never know it. This is not problematic, nor should it cause you or the patient any alarm unless the patient is preterm and experiencing contractions or rupture of membranes.

○ Primigravid patients will usually take longer to begin dilating and effacing. Many women will become upset and frustrated when they reach 38 or 39 weeks and have not begun dilating. Reassurance is key.

○ A good rule of thumb is that if you can insert one finger into the endocervical canal, the patient is 1 to 2 cm. Two fingers is 3 to 4 cm. Two fingers with room for a third is about 5 to 6 cm. Enough room for four fingers is 7 to 8 cm. Remember that active labor begins once the cervix has dilated to at least 5 cm (Figure 1.1).

CLINICAL PEARL: Never perform a digital exam prior to a speculum exam in a patient with suspected rupture of membranes.

Key Points . . .

- Each prenatal visit is an opportunity to provide screening, patient education, and anticipatory guidance.
- Listening for FHTs with a hand held Doppler is an expectation for all prenatal visits after 12 weeks.
- Never perform a digital exam on a gravid patient who presents with bleeding in the third trimester.
- Gravid patients who present in the second or third trimester with possible rupture of membranes need to have a sterile speculum exam prior to any other cervical manipulation.

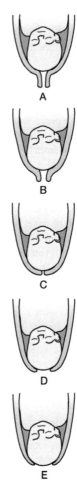

Figure 1.1   Stages of cervix dilation. (A) Not effaced, length of cervical canal is 4 cm; (B) partly effaced, length of cervical canal is 2 cm; (C) fully effaced; (D) dilated 3 cm; (E) dilated 8 cm.

References

1. Kilpatrick SJ, Papile L-A, Macones GA, eds. *Guidelines for Perinatal Care.* 8th ed. Elk Grove Village, IL: American Academy of Pediatrics; Washington, DC: American College of Obstetricians and Gynecologists; 2017. https://www.acog.org/Clinical%20Guidance%20and%20Publications/Guidelines%20for%20Perinatal%20Care.aspx

2. Gupta S, Roman AS. Imaging in obstetrics. In: DeCherney AH, Nathan L, Laufer N, Roman AS ed. *Current Diagnosis and Treatment: Obstetrics and Gynecology.* New York, NY: McGraw-Hill Medical; 2013:214–221.

3. Bernstein HB, VanBuren G. Normal pregnancy and prenatal care. In: DeCherney AH, Nathan L, Laufer N, Roman AS ed. *Current Diagnosis and Treatment: Obstetrics and Gynecology.* New York, NY: McGraw-Hill Medical; 2013:141–153.

4. Li D-K, Ferber JR, Odouli R, Quesenberry C. Use of nonsteroidal anti-inflammatory drugs during pregnancy and the risk of miscarriage. *Am J Obstet Gynecol.* 2018;219(3):275.e1–275.e8. doi:10.1016/j.ajog.2018.06.002

VAGINAL DISCHARGE

Do not hesitate to ask the nurse or medical assistant whether the patient's insurance dictates the use of a specific specimen collection system. Be prepared to have all of your equipment ready on the Mayo stand in the room with the patient. Once the patient is undressed and on the exam table, you do not want to have to leave the room to get a different specimen collection tube for a viral PCR, for example. Sometimes patients will complain of vaginal discharge or even a possible urinary tract infection (UTI) when they actually are experiencing a primary genital herpes outbreak; therefore, it is important to always perform an exam.

Differential Diagnosis

- Bacterial vaginosis
- Trichomoniasis
- Candidiasis
- Gonorrhea
- Chlamydia
- Mycoplasma
- Foreign body
- Atrophic vaginitis
- Herpes simplex virus

History

- Onset, duration, and timing: Ask when the LMP occurred and whether the patient uses tampons. Ask the patient whether the symptoms occur after intercourse, before menses, sporadically, or regularly. Some women will experience vaginitis after sexual intercourse, with the use of condoms, and/or with spermicides. Ask for how long the patient has experienced the discharge, and whether there is any odor. A fishy odor can be indicative of bacterial vaginosis or trichomoniasis. A musty or malodorous vaginal discharge can occur when a tampon has remained in the vagina for days to weeks after the menses has ceased. Has the patient recently taken antibiotics? Some women are more sensitive to antibiotics and will develop a vulvovaginitis due to yeast after the use of antibiotics. Recurrent candidiasis may occur in a patient with poorly controlled diabetes. A patient who is postmenopausal or taking anti-estrogen chemotherapy can develop atrophic vaginitis.

> **CLINICAL PEARL:** Pruritic vaginal discharge that occurs a few days to a week premenstrually is often due to overgrowth of lactobacillus secondary to increased estrogen. Women who use combined hormonal contraceptives will sometimes develop a vulvovaginal candidiasis due to the estrogen in the contraceptives.

- Provoking/alleviating factors: Does using over-the-counter antifungals help or make the symptoms worse? Does sexual intercourse make the symptoms worse? Does the patient notice any relationship between diet and symptoms?

> **CLINICAL PEARL:** Sexual activity can aggravate or cause a bacterial vaginosis in some women.

- Quality: Does the patient have any itching or burning? Is there discharge on the patient's underwear, or is it only just an odor? If there is actual discharge, what color is it? Is the discharge heavy enough that the patient requires a pantiliner?

> **CLINICAL PEARL:** Retained tampons can cause a profuse malodorous vaginal discharge. The foreign object can be easily removed with a ring forceps. However, if a patient is febrile and shows any signs of toxicity, a culture of the vagina is indicated, as is emergent management of the patient.

- Associated symptoms: Important associated symptoms would include fever, chills, pelvic pain, dysuria, dyspareunia, pruritus, vulvar pain, myalgias, fatigue, and abdominal pain. Fever, chills, and pelvic pain may indicate PID.

> **CLINICAL PEARL:** Patients with primary genital herpes will often experience a prodrome of fever, myalgias, and flu-like symptoms up to a week before the lesions occur.

Past Medical History and Review of Symptoms Specific to Complaint

- General: Recent infection that required antibiotics
- Endocrine: Diabetes mellitus; disease that would necessitate the use of glucocorticoids
- Infectious: History of STIs
- Rheumatologic: Disease that would necessitate the use of glucocorticoids
- Sexual: Ask about sexual partners, new products being used (lubricants, latex toys), anal–vaginal intercourse; placing foreign objects in the vagina can cause trauma and bacterial vaginosis, and retained tampons can cause toxic shock syndrome, a *Staphylococcal* sepsis; bacterial vaginosis is more common among women who have sex with women and women who receive oral sex; assess the patient's risk factors for STIs and PID

Social History

Ask about sexual practices including use of sexual toys.

Physical Examination

The physical examination in a patient with a chief complaint of vaginal discharge must include a pelvic examination. It can be tempting to treat the patient based on her symptoms, but antibiotic stewardship and good clinical practice mandate that a proper diagnosis be established prior to treatment. Table 1.11 provides a guide to common physical examination findings and their associated clinical conditions.

TABLE 1.11 Correlating Physical Exam Findings With Pathologic Conditions

Body or Organ System	Physical Exam Finding	Associated Clinical Condition
General appearance	Toxic appearing	Pelvic inflammatory disease, toxic shock syndrome
Vital signs	Fever	Pelvic inflammatory disease
	Tachycardia	Pelvic inflammatory disease
Abdomen	Tenderness	Pelvic inflammatory disease
Vulva and perineum	Vesicles and/or ulcerations	Genital herpes simplex
	Small fissures	Vulvovaginal candidiasis

(continued)

TABLE 1.11 Correlating Physical Exam Findings With Pathologic Conditions (*continued*)

Body or Organ System	Physical Exam Finding	Associated Clinical Condition
Vagina	Thick, white clumpy discharge ("cottage cheese appearance"); can have "fishy" smell	Vulvovaginal candidiasis
	Milky nonadherent discharge, "fishy" smell ↑with KOH	Bacterial vaginosis
	Greenish-yellow, frothy, bubbly discharge	*Trichomoniasis*
	Pale epithelium, loss of rugae	Atrophic vaginitis
	Retained foreign object	Bacterial vaginosis, trauma, toxic shock syndrome
Cervix	Mucopurulent cervical discharge	Chlamydia, gonorrhea, *Mycoplasma hominis*
	Cervical friability	Chlamydia, gonorrhea, herpes simplex, trichomoniasis, *Mycoplasma hominis*, malignancy
	Punctate and papilliform (strawberry cervix)	Trichomoniasis
Bimanual exam	Diffuse tenderness	Pelvic inflammatory disease
	"Chandelier sign"	Pelvic inflammatory disease

↑ elevated or increased. KOH, potassium hydroxide.

Diagnostic Plan

- Vaginal and cervical swabs: Use facility- and insurance-specific swabs for each test.
  - Evaluate for chlamydia, gonorrhea, *Mycoplasma hominis*, herpes simplex.
- Wet mount: Can be evaluated in clinic or sent to the lab, depending on the facility.
  - Evaluate for candidiasis, trichomoniasis, bacterial vaginosis. See Table 1.12 for a description of the findings in each of these conditions.
- Cytology (Pap test) and/or human papillomavirus (HPV) testing, if patient is due for testing
  - Evaluate for cervical dysplasia.

Initial Management

The management of vaginal discharge depends on the underlying etiology. Atrophic vaginitis (now called the *genitourinary syndrome of menopause*) is often seen in postmenopausal women who are not using exogenous estrogen.[1,2]

TABLE 1.12 Differentiating Vaginal Discharges

Clinical Condition	Organisms	Wet-Prep Findings	Clinical Findings
Bacterial vaginosis	*Gardnerella vaginalis, Mycoplasma hominis, Ureaplasm urealyticum, Bacteroides, Mobiluncus*	Clue cells	Positive whiff test, pH >4.5
Vulvovaginal candidiasis	*Candida albicans, Candida glabrata*	Pseudohyphae, budding yeast	Thick, white, cottage-cheese discharge
Trichomoniasis[a]	*Trichomonas vaginalis*	Motile trichomonads	Thick or thin, yellowish or green vaginal discharge, +/- cervical friability, pH can be >4.5

[a]Considered a sexually transmitted infection.

- Trichomoniasis: Metronidazole 2 g orally in a single dose or tinidazole 2 g orally in a single dose
  - Do not use vaginal metronidazole for trichomoniasis.
  - If resistance is suspected, may use metronidazole 2 g orally for 7 days.
  - Pregnant women should be treated with metronidazole as trichomoniasis is associated with preterm rupture of membranes.
  - Trichomoniasis is a nonreportable STI, but partners of affected patients must be treated.
  - Remember to warn the patient of the disulfuram-like effect so she must abstain from using alcohol during the course of treatment.
- Gonorrhea: Ceftriaxone 250 mg intramuscularly (IM) with azithromycin 1 g × 1 day
- Chlamydia: Doxycycline 100 mg orally twice a day for 7 days or azithromycin 1 g orally × 1 day
- *Mycoplasma hominis*: Resistance to tetracycline and macrolides are high; can use a quinolone
- Vulvovaginal candidiasis: Oral fluconazole 150 mg (× 1, or for 3 consecutive days); vaginal clotrimazole or miconazole per package instructions
- Bacterial vaginosis: Metronidazole 500 mg orally twice a day for 7 days
  - Can also use metronidazole vaginal gel 0.75% one applicatorful once daily for 5 days.
  - Can use clindamycin vaginal cream 2% one full applicatorful at bedtime for 7 days.
- Herpes simplex virus: Acyclovir, valcyclovir, famciclovir; treatment regimens vary according to primary infection, recurrent, or episodic

- Atrophic vaginitis (genitourinary syndrome of menopause): Vaginal estrogen, intravaginal dehydroepiandrosterone (DHEA), ospemifene (a selective estrogen receptor modulator [SERM] with conjugated equine estrogen), or laser therapy

Key Points . . .

- Always perform a pelvic exam on a woman with a chief complaint of vaginal discharge. You must rule out retained foreign objects, trauma, and STIs.
- Some STIs are reportable to local health departments, such as chlamydia and gonorrhea.
- Trichomoniasis is a sexually transmitted disease, so partners need to be treated. However, it is not reportable to local or state health departments.
- Recurrent candidal vaginitis can be a sign of underlying diabetes, HIV, or the presence of a resistant species.
- Atrophic vaginitis in the absence of vasomotor symptoms should be treated with vaginal preparations.

References

1. Workowski KA, Bolan GA. 2015 sexually transmitted diseases guidelines. *MMWR Recomm Rep*. 2015;64(3):1–140. https://www.cdc.gov/std/tg2015/tg-2015-print.pdf
2. American College of Obstetricians and Gynecologists. ACOG Practice Bulletin No. 72: Vaginitis. https://www.acog.org/Clinical-Guidance-and-Publications/Practice-Bulletins/Committee-on-Practice-Bulletins-Gynecology/Vaginitis. Reaffirmed 2019.

2

Common Disease Entities in Gynecology

AMENORRHEA

Etiology[1]

- *Primary amenorrhea* is defined as the lack of menarche by age 13 in a young woman without breast development, or 15 in a woman with breast development.
- Secondary amenorrhea is the absence of menses for longer than 3 months in females with a history of regular menses, or 6 months in females with a history of irregular menses.

Epidemiology[1]

- The most common cause of primary amenorrhea is chromosomal abnormalities resulting in gonadal dysgenesis or Müellerian agenesis.
- The most common cause of secondary amenorrhea in a patient of reproductive age is pregnancy.
- The second most common cause is functional hypothalamic amenorrhea.
- Common underlying factors associated with functional hypothalamic amenorrhea are anorexia, excessive exercise, and emotional stress, but a specific precipitating factor is often not found.

Clinical Presentation

- Lack of menses as described earlier

Diagnosis

- The diagnosis of primary amenorrhea and secondary amenorrhea relies on patient history.
- It is important to distinguish oligomenorrhea from secondary amenorrhea.

- Determining the underlying etiology, however, requires further investigation with laboratory tests and imaging. See the section "Missed Menses/Amenorrhea" in Chapter 1, Common Presentations in Obstetrics and Gynecology.

Management

- The management of amenorrhea largely depends on its underlying etiology.
- Women without gonadal dysgenesis will need to use progestin therapy to protect the endometrium.
- Combination oral contraceptives or other hormonal options can be used in patients who do not have contraindications.
- Women who do not wish to take daily combined contraception can take progestin for 10 days every 3 to 4 months to induce a withdrawal bleed to protect the endometrium.
- Women with secondary amenorrhea who wish to conceive should be referred to a reproductive endocrinologist and be advised to begin folic acid supplementation.

> **CLINICAL PEARL:** Any woman of reproductive age who presents with amenorrhea or a missed menses must be ruled out for pregnancy.

REFERENCE

1. Simon A, Chang WY, DeCherney AH. Amenorrhea. In: DeCherney AH, Nathan L, Laufer N, et al., ed. *Current Diagnosis and Treatment: Obstetrics and Gynecology.* New York, NY: McGraw-Hill Medical; 2013:889–899.

ANTIPHOSPHOLIPID SYNDROME

Etiology[1]

- Antiphospholipid antibodies include lupus anticoagulant, anticardiolipin, and anti-beta-2 glycoprotein I.
- Antiphospholipid antibody syndrome can occur in patients with only one antibody, but some patients will have all the antibodies.
- Beta-2 glycoprotein I is involved in fibrinolysis and coagulation.
- Antiphospholipid antibody syndrome is linked to venous, arterial, and microvascular thrombotic events as well as fetal loss and autoimmune thrombocytopenia.
- Antiphospholipid antibody syndrome may be associated with intrauterine growth restriction, placental insufficiency, preeclampsia, and preterm deliveries.

Epidemiology[1]

- About 2% of venous thrombosis patients will test positive for antibodies to lupus anticoagulant.
- About 25% of venous thrombosis in patients who have antiphospholipid antibody syndrome occurs during pregnancy or postpartum.

Clinical Presentation[1]

- Patients with antiphospholipid antibody syndrome will have a history of any of the following:
  - Venous or arterial thrombosis
  - One or more episodes of a fetal demise after 10 weeks' gestation
  - One or more preterm deliveries of a chromosomally normal fetus prior to 34 weeks' gestation due to either preeclampsia or placental insufficiency
  - At least three consecutive early pregnancy losses before 10 weeks' gestation without maternal, paternal, or fetal chromosomal abnormalities

Diagnosis[1,2]

- Nonpregnant, pregnant, and postpartum patients who experience a venous thromboembolic event (VTE) should have laboratory testing for antiphospholipid antibody syndrome
- Antiphospholipid antibody syndrome can be tested by the following:
  - Presence of lupus anticoagulant on two different occasions with at least 12 weeks between tests
- Presence of medium to high titers of anticardiolipin antibody (immunoglobulin G [IgG] or immunoglobulin M [IgM]) on two different occasions with at least 12 weeks between tests
- Presence of anti-beta-2 glycoprotein I (IgG or IgM) on two different occasions with at least 12 weeks between tests
- Lupus anticoagulant is associated with more clinical events than anticardiolipin antibody and anti-beta-2 glycoprotein I

Management[1,2]

- Prophylactic anticoagulation should be considered in women with a history of a thrombotic event (see the section "Venous Thromboembolism" in Chapter 3, Common Disease Entities in Obstetrics).
- The use of low-dose aspirin to prevent adverse pregnancy outcomes in patients with antiphospholipid syndrome is controversial.

REFERENCES

1. American College of Obstetricians and Gynecologists. ACOG practice bulletin no. 132. Antiphospholipid syndrome. https://www.acog.org/Clinical-Guidance-and-Publications/Practice-Bulletins/Committee-on-Practice-Bulletins-Obstetrics/Antiphospholipid-Syndrome. Reaffirmed 2017.
2. Garcia D, Erkan D. Diagnosis and management of the antiphospholipid antibody syndrome. *N Engl J Med*. 2018. 378(21):2010–2021. doi:10.1056/NEJMra1705454

Bartholin Cyst and Abscess

Etiology
- The Bartholin glands are two pea-sized glands that produce mucus and help with vaginal lubrication.
- Occasionally, the glands become blocked and the fluid cannot drain, resulting in cyst formation.
- A Bartholin gland abscess occurs when the cyst or gland becomes infected.
- *Escherichia coli* is the most common organism isolated from abscesses.

Epidemiology
- Bartholin cysts and abscesses are responsible for approximately 2% of gynecologic visits annually.[1]
- Most women with a Bartholin cyst or abscess will be in their 20s.[2]
- Women 40 years and older who present with a Bartholin gland issue should undergo biopsy.

Clinical Presentation
- Patients will present with a "bulge" or "mass" that they will often say is in their vagina.
- Most patients will have some level of discomfort, depending on whether they have a cyst or an abscess.
- Patients with an abscess will have considerable pain.
- An atypical-appearing Bartholin mass should be evaluated for malignancy.

Diagnosis
- Diagnosis is established by physical examination (Figure 2.1)

Management[1,2]
- Abscesses and cysts must be incised and drained followed by placement of a Word catheter or gauze.
- See the section "Bartholin Gland Cyst and Abscess" in Chapter 6, Common Procedures in Gynecology.
- Recurrent cysts and abscesses may require marsupialization, a surgical procedure that removes the entire gland.
- Antibiotics may be used but evidence is lacking regarding optimal antimicrobial dosing and duration.
- If you choose to use an antimicrobial, remember that *E. coli* is the most common organism and that *Neisseria gonorrhoeae* and *Chlamydia trachomatis* are rarely causative organisms.

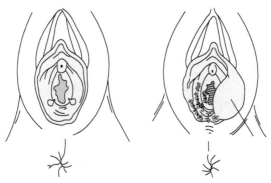

Figure **2.1** Illustration showing (left) Bartholin glands and (right) Bartholin cyst.
Source: From Secor RM, Fantasia HC. *Fast Facts About the Gynecologic Exam.* 2nd ed. New York, NY: Springer Publishing Company; 2018:31.

References

1. Quinn A. Bartholin gland diseases, treatment, and management. In: Schraga ED, ed. *Medscape.* https://emedicine.medscape.com/article/777112-treatment. Updated August 10, 2017.
2. Shlamovitz GZ. Bartholin abscess drainage. In: Isaacs C, ed. *Medscape.* https://emedicine.medscape.com/article/80260-overview#a8. Updated January 8, 2019.

Breast Abscess

Etiology
- Breast abscesses are a complication of mastitis and are usually caused by *Staphylococcus aureus.*

Epidemiology
- Fewer than 1% of breastfeeding women will develop a breast abscess.[1]
- Risk factors include tobacco use, incomplete emptying of the breast, maternal age greater than 30 years, and primiparity.

Clinical Presentation
- Breast abscesses present as a painful, erythematous, fluctuant breast mass accompanied by fever, chills, and malaise.
- Often there is a recent history of mastitis.

Diagnosis

- The diagnosis can sometimes be made by physical examination, but breast ultrasonography helps to differentiate mastitis from an abscess.

Management[2]

- Abscesses must be drained. Needle aspiration, with or without ultrasound guidance, of abscesses smaller than 3 cm can offer cosmetic benefits.
- Percutaneous catheter placement can be considered in patients with abscesses larger than 3 cm.
- Abscesses larger than 5 cm should be surgically incised and drained.
- Abscesses that are multiloculated, look as if they may rupture the skin, or are unresponsive to antibiotics should be surgically incised and drained.
- In patients in whom methicillin-resistant *Staphylococcus aureus* (MRSA) is suspected, a culture is recommended.
- Antimicrobial selection includes dicloxacillin, cephalexin, clindamycin, or trimethoprim/sulfamethoxazole (TMP/SMX).
- Clindamycin and TMP/SMX can be used if MRSA is suspected or confirmed.
- If nipple retraction is present, or the abscess is subareolar, metronidazole should be added to the antimicrobial of choice.
- Women should be encouraged to continue breastfeeding or to use a breast pump.

CLINICAL PEARL: Patients who do not respond to incision and drainage (I&D) and antimicrobial therapy must be ruled out for Paget's disease of the breast or inflammatory breast cancer.

REFERENCES

1. Dener C, Inan A. Breast abscesses in lactating women. *World J Surg.* 2003;27(2): 130–133. doi:10.1007/s00268-002-6563-6
2. Lam E, Chan T, Wiseman SM. Breast abscess: evidence-based management recommendations. *Expert Rev Anti Infect Ther.* 2014;12(7):753–762. doi:10 .1586/14787210.2014.913982

BREAST CANCER

Etiology[1]

- Risk factors for breast cancer include *BRCA* mutations, which account for approximately 10% of all breast cancer; other risk factors include increasing age, obesity, age greater than 30 at first birth, and menarche before age 13 years.

TABLE **2.1** Overview of Breast Cancer Subtypes

Subtype	Immunohistochemistry	Prognosis	Notes
Luminal A	ER positive PR positive HER2 negative	Good	The most common subtype. Responsive to hormone therapies such as SERMs and AIs.
Luminal B	ER positive PR positive HER2 positive or negative	Fair	Tend to be of higher grade. Tend to recur more frequently than luminal A.
HER2 over-expression	ER negative PR negative HER2 positive	Poor	Not all tumors respond to anti-HER2 monoclonal antibodies. Resistance to treatment can occur with certain chemotherapies.
Basal (often called *triple negative*)	ER negative PR negative HER2 negative	Poor	Not amenable to hormone therapy or HER2 therapy. Specific targeted therapies are under investigation.

AIs, aromatase inhibitors; ER, estrogen-receptor; HER2, human epidermal growth factor type 2; PR, progesterone; SERMs, selective estrogen receptor modulators.

- Different histologies are associated with various risk factors.
- Immunohistochemical markers help to stratify patients for treatment options and prognosis, along with staging of disease (Table 2.1).
- Infiltrating ductal carcinoma (IDC) is the most common histologic type (up to 80%), followed by invasive lobular (8%).
- Ductal carcinoma in situ (DCIS) is a heterogeneous group of noninfiltrating, localized malignancies that are subcategorized based on morphology, anatomical location, and cytological features.
- Some infiltrating ductal carcinomas will have the presence of DCIS as well.
- Infiltrating lobular carcinomas (ILC) occur more frequently in postmenopausal women and tend to occur in both breasts.
- Almost all ILCs are hormone-receptor positive.
- Inflammatory breast cancers are less common but tend to be much more aggressive and offer a worse prognosis.

Epidemiology[1,2]

- In the United States, more women will be diagnosed with breast cancer than any other malignancy.
- One in eight women will be diagnosed with some form of breast cancer during her lifetime.
- Black women in the United States are generally diagnosed at a later stage and have decreased life expectancy compared with non-Hispanic Whites.

Clinical Presentation[1,3]

- Approximately 30% of women will present with a palpable breast mass.
- The typical description of a hard, immobile mass with irregular borders can be difficult to qualify on physical exam, thus, any new mass requires evaluation.
- Breast lesions may be found on screening mammograms.
- Advanced disease can present with axillary lymphadenopathy and breast distortion.
- Inflammatory breast cancer presents with breast skin changes, such as dimpling or an orange-peel appearance to the breast, that can mimic mastitis or an abscess and, as such, is always in the differential diagnosis of a patient with mastitis or abscess.

Diagnosis

- Certain breast cancers have typical mammographic or ultrasonic findings.
- Spiculation, pleomorphic microcalcifications, and anatomic distortion are common mammographic findings of breast cancer.
- Irregular shape, hypoechoic echotexture, and posterior acoustic shadowing are common sonographic findings in breast malignancies.
- Ultrasound is also used to assess the axilla for abnormal lymph nodes.
- The American College of Radiology utilizes the Breast Imaging-Reporting and Data System (BI-RADS) to classify mammogram and ultrasound findings. Images are graded from 0 to 6. Please see www.acr.org/-/media/ACR/Files/RADS/BI-RADS/BIRADS-Reference-Card.pdf for more information.
- Breast MRI can be used to further assess extent of disease and is often utilized in presurgical planning of biopsy-proven breast cancer.
- Diagnosis is dependent upon tissue analysis.
- Depending on the clinical scenario, tissue can be obtained via excisional biopsy, ultrasound-guided core-needle biopsy, stereotactic biopsy, or MRI-guided biopsy.

Management[1,4]

- The management of breast cancer is dependent on multiple factors, including age of patient, size of lesion, presence of recurrent disease, extent of disease, histologic type, and patient preference.
- Early-stage breast cancer can be managed surgically with mastectomy or lumpectomy followed by radiation therapy.
- Medical options depend on estrogen and progesterone receptor status and human epidermal growth factor type 2 (HER2) expression.
- Most breast cancers are graded by their level of cellular differentiation, responsiveness to estrogen and progesterone, and expression of HER2.

- Malignancies that are estrogen and progesterone receptor positive tend to grow more rapidly but can be treated with selective estrogen receptor modulators (SERMs) and aromatase inhibitors (AIs).
  - SERMS are generally used in patients who are premenopausal or perimenopausal for their positive effects on bone.
  - AIs are generally used in postmenopausal patients.
  - Current evidence recommends 5 years of a SERM in premenopausal women followed by 5 years of an AI.
  - AIs block estrogen conversion so women who take an AI must have their bone density evaluated on a regular basis.
- Malignancies that are HER2 positive also tend to grow more rapidly but can be treated with drugs that block the HER2 protein, such as pertuzumab and trastuzamab. However, not all HER2 positive breast cancers respond to anti-HER2 monoclonal antibodies.
- Patients with locally advanced breast cancer are usually offered presurgical chemotherapy (referred to as *neoadjuvant*) followed by surgical resection.
- Postsurgical chemotherapy (referred to as *adjuvant* and includes endocrine therapy) depends on the histology, hormone receptor status, and HER2 expression of the primary tumor.

> **CLINICAL PEARL:** Women with a history of estrogen-receptor-positive breast cancer cannot use systemic hormones. Survivorship counseling and medical management must include evidence-based nonhormonal alternatives.

REFERENCES

1. American Cancer Society. *Breast Cancer Facts & Figures 2017–2018.* Atlanta, GA: Author; 2017. https://www.cancer.org/content/dam/cancer-org/research/cancer-facts-and-statistics/breast-cancer-facts-and-figures/breast-cancer-facts-and-figures-2017-2018.pdf.
2. Torre LA, Bray F, Siegel RL, et al. Global cancer statistics, 2012. *CA Cancer J Clin.* 2015;65(2):87–108. doi:10.3322/caac.21262
3. Esserman LJ, Shieh Y, Rutgers EJ, et al. Impact of mammographic screening on the detection of good and poor prognosis breast cancers. *Breast Cancer Res Treat.* 2011;130(3):725–734. doi:10.1007/s10549-011-1748-z
4. National Cancer Institute. Breast Cancer Treatment (PDQ®)–Health Professional Version. https://www.cancer.gov/types/breast/hp/breast-treatment-pdq. Updated June 20, 2019.

CERVICAL CANCER

Etiology[1]

- Over 99% of cervical cancer is caused by oncogenic human papillomavirus (HPV) subtypes.
- HPV attaches to and infects the cervical basal cells, usually in the transformation zone.
- It can take 10 to 20 years after exposure to oncogenic HPV to undergo malignant transformation.

Epidemiology[2]

- About 12,500 women are diagnosed with cervical cancer each year, and rates continue to decline due to Pap testing.
  - It is possible that with HPV immunization, that number will decline even further.
- Early age at sexual activity, multiple sexual partners, smoking, and immunodeficiency are major risk factors.

Clinical Presentation

- Cervical cancer can be asymptomatic.
- In later disease, women can present with irregular uterine bleeding and postcoital bleeding.

Diagnosis

- Diagnosis is made by biopsy.
- Staging of disease uses the histological findings of biopsy, plus the size of the mass, uterine size, presence of parametrial and vaginal extension, presence of inguinal and/or supraclavicular lymph nodes, and careful right upper quadrant palpation.
- A rectovaginal exam is necessary to adequately assess the pelvis.
- Sometimes cystoscopy and proctosigmoidoscopy are used to visualize the respective areas.
- Other ancillary testing includes a complete blood count (CBC), chemistry panel, liver enzymes, chest x-ray, and CT of the pelvis and abdomen.
- MRI and PET scans can be ordered as an alternative to CT; PET scanning is recommended for all patients at stage 1B2 or higher.
- Staging of disease follows Fédération Internationale de Gynécologie et d'Obstétrique (FIGO) and TNM classifications.[3]
- Cervical cancer can manifest with lymphatic spread to the peritoneum, supraclavicular nodes, mediastinal nodes, and para-aortic nodes.[3]
- Metastatic disease can occur in the lung, the liver, and bone.[3]
- An overview of the TNM classification is as follows:[3]
  - TX: Primary tumor cannot be assessed
  - T0: No evidence of a primary tumor

- Tis: Carcinoma in situ
- T1: Carcinoma confined to the cervix
- T2: Carcinoma invasion beyond the uterus that does not extend to pelvic walls or lower one third of vagina
- T3: Tumor extends to the pelvic wall and/or the lower one third of the vagina and/or causes hydronephrosis
- T4: Tumor invades bladder mucosa or rectum and/or extends beyond the pelvis
- NX: Lymph nodes cannot be assessed
- N0: No regional lymph node metastasis
- N1: Regional lymph node metastasis is present
- M0: No distant metastasis
- M1: Distant metastasis is present
- The FIGO classification is as follows:[3]
  - Stage 0: Carcinoma in situ
  - Stage I: Carcinoma confined to the cervix
  - Stage II: Carcinoma extends beyond the cervix but not to the pelvic wall or lower one third of the vagina
  - Stage III: Tumor extends beyond the cervix to the pelvic wall and/or lower one third of the vagina and/or causes hydronephrosis or a non-functioning kidney
  - Stage IV: Tumor invades the bladder mucosa and/or rectum and/or extends beyond the pelvis
  - Both the FIGO and TNM classifications are subdivided based on tumor size and stromal and parametrial invasion

Management[4]

- The management of cervical cancer largely depends upon the staging of disease.
- Stage 0 disease can be managed with laser ablation or loop excision.
- Earlier disease can be managed operatively with hysterectomy.
  - Surgical decisions in early disease must consider the patient's desire to preserve fertility.
- In patients with stage Ia1 disease, lymph node dissection is not required only if the depth of the tumor's invasion is less than 3 mm and no lymphovascular invasion is found.
- In patients with Ia2, Ib, or IIa disease, options include external beam radiation and brachytherapy or complete hysterectomy with bilateral pelvic lymphadenectomy.
- Later stage options include brachytherapy, external beam radiation therapy, lymphadenectomy, and platinum-based chemotherapy regimens.
- Other systemic chemotherapeutic options include 5-fluorouracil (5-FU), docetaxel, gemcitabine, mitomycin, irinotecan, topotecan, pemetrexed, vinorelbine, and bevacizumab.

References

1. Centers for Disease Control and Prevention. Introduction to HPV. https://www.cdc.gov/cancer/knowledge/provider-education/hpv/introduction.htm
2. United States Cancer Statistics Working Group. *United States Cancer Statistics: 1999–2014 Incidence and Mortality Web-Based Report*. Atlanta, GA: Department of Health and Human Services, Centers for Disease Control and Prevention, and National Cancer Institute; 2017.
3. Boardman CH. Cervical cancer staging. In: Sonoda Y, ed. *Medscape*. https://emedicine.medscape.com/article/2006486-overview. Updated April 26, 2019.
4. Boardman CH. Cervical cancer treatment and management. In: Huh WK, ed. *Medscape*. https://emedicine.medscape.com/article/253513-treatment. Updated February 12, 2019.

CERVICAL DYSPLASIA

Etiology

- *Cervical dysplasia* is a term used to describe lesions of the cervix that are precancerous.
- The vast majority of cervical dysplasia or cervical intraepithelial neoplasia (CIN) are caused by HPV.
- Cervical intraepithelial lesions are categorized into two separate entities: low-grade and high-grade lesions.
    - CIN I is considered a low-grade squamous intraepithelial lesion (LSIL), usually caused by low-risk HPV subtypes such as 6 and 11.
    - CIN 2 tissue samples are tested for p16 immunostaining. CIN 2 with negative p16 are LSIL, and CIN2 with positive p16 are high-grade squamous intraepithelial lesions (HSIL).
    - CIN 3 is an HSIL, caused by high-risk HPV subtypes such as 16 and 18.

Epidemiology

- Approximately 80% of women undergoing Pap testing will test positive for a low- or high-risk lesion.[1]
- Vaccination is decreasing the incidence of CIN in younger women.
- Adults can receive the 9-valent HPV vaccine up until age 45 years.

Clinical Presentation

- Low-grade and high-grade lesions are asymptomatic.
- Possible lesions are found on Pap testing and/or HPV test screening.

Diagnosis

- Diagnosis is confirmed with colposcopy, biopsy, and an endocervical curettage.
- Classic colposcopic findings of an LSIL are acetopositive lesions with fine vascular punctuation and homogenous mosaicism.

- Classic colposcopic findings in HSIL are acetopositive lesions with sharp borders, coarse mosaicism, neovascularization, and cervical friability.

Management[2]

- Management of cervical dysplasia largely depends on a woman's risk factors and presence or absence of oncogenic, high-risk HPV subtypes.
- Pap testing should not begin until age 21.
- Pap testing and HPV testing (called *co-testing*) is not recommended for women 21 to 29 years.
- Women 30 to 65 years can undergo screening with cytology alone every 3 years, high-risk HPV testing alone every 5 years, or high-risk HPV with cytology every 5 years.
- Women age 30 years or more who test positive for a high-risk HPV subtype should undergo colposcopy even if she does not have an LSIL or HSIL on Pap testing.
- Women 25 and over with a positive HPV and either LSIL or HSIL should undergo colposcopy and biopsy.
- Women age 21 to 24 with atypical squamous cells of undetermined significance (ASC-US) or LSIL should have a repeat Pap test in 1 year.
- Women with biopsy-proven HSIL should undergo lesion excision with loop electrosurgical excision procedure (LEEP) or cone biopsy unless she is pregnant.
- Biopsy in pregnant women is deferred until postpartum.
  - ○ Colposcopy without biopsy can be performed with adequate documentation of visual findings with repeat testing to be completed postpartum.

REFERENCES

1. Centers for Disease Control and Prevention. Introduction to PHV. https://www.cdc.gov/cancer/knowledge/provider-education/hpv/introduction.htm
2. Massad LS, Einstein MH, Huh WKet al. 2012 updated consensus guidelines for the management of abnormal cervical cancer screening tests and cancer precursors. *J Low Genit Tract Dis.* 2012;17(5) (suppl 1):S1–S27. doi:10.1097/LGT.0b013e318287d329

CERVICITIS

Etiology[1]

- Cervicitis can be divided into infectious and noninfectious etiologies.
- Infectious etiologies are the most common, and are usually due to sexually transmitted infections (STIs) such as chlamydia, gonorrhea, and herpes simplex.
  - ○ Trichomoniasis can also cause cervicitis.
  - ○ An increase in *Mycoplasma genitalium* incidence is being identified.

- Noninfectious causes include brachytherapy, chemical irritation, local trauma, and systemic disease such as Behçet disease.

Epidemiology[2]

- The epidemiology of cervicitis includes rates for chlamydia and gonorrhea infections.
- In 2016, a total of 1,598,354, or a rate of 497.3 cases per 100,000 population were identified, an increase of 4.7% compared with the rate in 2015.
- In 2016, 468,514 gonorrhea cases were reported, for a rate of 145.8 cases per 100,000 population, an increase of 18.5% from 2015.
- Drug-resistant strains of gonorrhea are increasing in incidence.

Clinical Presentation

- Many women are symptomatic.
- Some women will complain of postcoital bleeding, dyspareunia, dysuria, and vaginal discharge.
- On physical exam, there will be purulent or mucopurulent cervical discharge from the os.
  - The cervix can be friable, and some women will have mild tenderness when the cervix is palpated and moved (referred to as *cervical motion tenderness* or the *chandelier sign*)
- Punctate hemorrhages on the cervix can make the cervix appear as if it were a strawberry.
  - This is a classic finding for trichomoniasis cervicitis.
- Ulcerations or vesicles on the cervix are found with herpes simplex cervicitis.

Diagnosis

- Diagnosis can be confirmed with nucleic acid amplification testing (NAAT) for *Neisseria gonorrhoeae*, *Chlamydia trachomatis*, and *Trichomonas vaginalis*.
- Viral culture can be obtained if herpes is suspected, but if ulcers are present, it is prudent to also check serology for syphilis.
- There are no current recommendations for testing for *Mycoplasma vaginalis*.

Management[3]

- The management of infectious cervicitis depends on first ruling out the presence of pelvic inflammatory disease.
- Once ruled out, empiric treatment can be started.
- Women younger than 25 years of age or who are at high risk for STIs should be treated for presumptive chlamydia.
- The Centers for Disease Control and Prevention recommends that chlamydia be treated with azithromycin 1 g by mouth one time, or doxycycline 100 mg twice a day by mouth for 7 days if the patient is unable to tolerate azithromycin.

- Gonorrhea should be treated with ceftriaxone 250 mg intramuscularly for 1 day WITH azithromycin 1 g × 1 day or doxycycline 100 mg twice a day for 7 days.
- Treatment of *Monochoria vaginalis* can be accomplished with azithromycin 1 g × 1 day.
- The treatment for trichomoniasis is metronidazole or tinidazole 2 g × 1 day by mouth
  - Do not use vaginal metronidazole gels or creams for trichomoniasis.
- Trichomoniasis, chlamydia, gonorrhea, and herpes are STIs so patient education must include ways to decrease transmission, prevent infections, and underscore the importance of sexual partners being treated.

References

1. Ollendorff AT. Cervicitis. In: Karjane NW, ed. *Medscape*. https://emedicine.medscape.com/article/253402-overview. Updated February 9, 2017.
2. Centers for Disease Control and Prevention. *Sexually Transmitted Disease Surveillance 2016*. Atlanta, GA: U.S. Department of Health and Human Services; 2017. https://www.cdc.gov/std/stats16/CDC_2016_STDS_Report-for508WebSep 21_2017_1644.pdf
3. Centers for Disease Control and Prevention. 2015 sexually transmitted diseases treatment guidelines. 2015. https://www.cdc.gov/std/tg2015/default.htm

Dysmenorrhea

Etiology

- Primary dysmenorrhea is painful menses that occurs in the absence of known pathology, usually in the first 6 months of menarche.
- The pathophysiology of primary dysmenorrhea is increasing prostaglandin secretion during the menstrual cycle.
  - Prostaglandins are potent vasoconstrictors and myometrial stimulators.
- Secondary dysmenorrhea is painful menses that occurs due to an underlying pathology such as endometriosis.
- Prostaglandins likely play a role in the pathophysiology of secondary dysmenorrhea, but by definition, secondary dysmenorrhea occurs in the presence of an underlying pathology that is usually responsible for the painful menses.

Epidemiology

- About 50% of menstruating women will experience dysmenorrhea.[1]

Clinical Presentation

- Patients will present with complaints of pelvic pain during menses.
- Patients may also experience low-back pain, pelvic bloating, and upper leg/thigh pain.

Diagnosis

- A thorough history and physical examination will help narrow the differential diagnosis.
- Primary dysmenorrhea is a clinical diagnosis, thus, interventional procedures are rarely indicated.
- Always ask the patient about age at menarche, cycle length and duration, other associated symptoms, gravida and para status, history of pelvic infections or surgeries, and history of sexual abuse or assault.
- The physical exam should include all aspects of the pelvic exam with careful attention to signs of trauma, vaginal discharge, uterine size and mobility, adnexal masses and tenderness, cervical motion tenderness and lesions, and masses or tenderness along the uterosacral ligaments.
- A pelvic ultrasound may show leiomyoma, adnexal masses, and foreign objects in the uterus (e.g., an intrauterine system [IUS])
- If the pelvic ultrasound is nondiagnostic, a diagnostic laparoscopy should be considered.

Management

- The initial management of primary dysmenorrhea is administration of nonsteroidal anti-inflammatory drugs (NSAIDS).
- If NSAIDS do not relieve the symptoms, many patients obtain relief with combination estrogen and progestin contraception.
- Treatment of secondary dysmenorrhea depends on the underlying etiology.
- There is no role for opioids in the management of dysmenorrhea.

REFERENCE

1. Iacovides S, Avidon I, Baker FC. What we know about primary dysmenorrhea today: a critical review. *Hum Reprod Update*. 2015;21(6):762–778. doi:10.1093/humupd/dmv039

ENDOMETRIAL CANCER

Etiology

- Unopposed exogenous or endogenous estrogen is the largest risk factor.
- Obesity, use of exogenous unopposed estrogen, chronic unintentional anovulation, nulliparity, Lynch syndrome (also known as *hereditary nonpolyposis colorectal cancer [HNPCC]*), and tamoxifen use are all risk factors.
- Adenocarcinoma is the most common histological type of uterine cancer.

- Although postmenopausal bleeding is often caused by benign atrophic conditions, all women are presumed to have malignancy until tissue sampling proves otherwise unless the endometrial thickness is less than 4 mm.

Epidemiology[1]

- Endometrial cancer is the most common gynecologic malignancy in the United States.
- The average age at diagnosis is 62 years but is trending to lower ages at diagnosis.

Clinical Presentation[2–4]

- The most common presenting symptom is abnormal uterine bleeding.
- Occasionally, the presence of atypical glandular cells or adenocarcinoma are found viaroutine Pap testing.
- In women over age 40, the presence of endometrial cells on a Pap test should prompt further workup if the patient is at risk for endometrial cancer.
- Sometimes endometrial hyperplasia and cancer are found incidentally on pelvic ultrasound, and sometimes are an incidental finding at hysterectomy.

Diagnosis[2–4]

- A transvaginal pelvic ultrasound with a measurement of the endometrial stripe (EMS) is a necessary first step.
- American College of Obstetricians and Gynecologists (ACOG) recommends that an EMS larger than 4 mm in a postmenopausal woman requires endometrial tissue sampling[5]
- An endometrial biopsy (EMB), if performed correctly, is accomplished in the office without need for anesthesia.
- A dilation and curettage, with or without hysteroscopy, is sometimes performed in lieu of the EMB if patients cannot tolerate the in-office procedure, or if bleeding is too heavy.
- Staging of disease uses the FIGO/TNM system
  - ○ Low risk:
    - Stage IA
      - Grade 1 confined to endometrium
  - ○ Intermediate risk:
    - Stage 1A or 1B with invasion into the myometrium
    - Stage II
  - ○ High risk:
    - Stage III or higher, regardless of histology

Management[2–4]

- Management depends on the staging of disease, but prompt referral to a gynecologic oncologist is recommended.
- Type I cancers are estrogen dependent and are associated with a good prognosis.[3]

- Type II cancers are nonestrogen dependent and are generally associated with a poor prognosis.[3]
- Surgical management is accomplished via hysterectomy and bilateral salpingo-oopherectomy and lymph node dissection.
- Biomarkers are being explored as possible prognosticators.
- Chemotherapy is usually carboplatin and paclitaxel.
  - Stage 1A grade 1 in women who wish to preserve fertility can use progestin therapy, but a high risk of recurrence occurs; therefore, patients should have hysterectomy and bilateral salpingo-oopherectomy (BSO) as soon as childbearing has been completed.
  - Intermediate risk: Surgery, followed by postoperative radiation therapy: Some gynecologic oncologists will offer adjuvant chemotherapy for higher risk of disease.
  - High risk: Surgery, chemotherapy, maybe radiation therapy: Options for chemotherapy are dependent on histology, invasion, and other risk factors.

REFERENCES

1. National Cancer Institute. Cancer stat facts: uterine cancer. http://seer.cancer.gov/statfacts/html/corp.html
2. Fleming ND, Dorigo O. Premalignant and malignant disorders of the uterine corpus. In: DeCherney AH, Nathan L, Laufer N, Roman AS, ed. *Current Diagnosis and Treatment: Obstetrics and Gynecology*. New York, NY: McGraw-Hill Medical; 2013:833–847.
3. Hacker NF. Uterine corpus cancer. In: Hacker NF, Gambone JC, Hobel CJ, eds. *Hacker and Moore's Essentials of Obstetrics and Gynecology*. 6th ed. Philadelphia, PA: Saunders/Elsevier; 2016:457–464.
4. SGO Clinical Practice Endometrial Cancer Working Group. Endometrial cancer: a review and current management strategies: part II. *Gynecol Onc*. 2014;134:393–402.
5. American College of Obstetricians and Gynecologists. Practice bulletin no. 149. Endometrial cancer. https://www.acog.org/Clinical-Guidance-and-Publications/Practice-Bulletins/Committee-on-Practice-Bulletins-Gynecology/Endometrial-Cancer. Reaffirmed 2017.

ENDOMETRIOSIS

Etiology[1,2]

- Endometriosis is the presence of endometrial glands and stroma outside of the uterus that can cause significant pelvic pain, dysmenorrhea, dyspareunia, dyschezia, and infertility, depending upon the location of the implants,
- Endometriosis is a nonmalignant estrogen-dependent process.

Epidemiology[1,2]

- Incidence ranges from 1% to 7%
- Protective factors include multiparity and prolonged lactation
- Risk factors include early menarche and excess estrogen exposure

Clinical Presentation

- Some women with endometriosis are asymptomatic and implants are found incidentally during a pelvic surgery.
- The typical presentation in symptomatic women is chronic pelvic pain, dysmenorrhea, dyspareunia, and infertility.
- Patients with posterior implants may experience dyschezia.

Diagnosis

- The diagnosis is made by direct visualization of endometriotic implants during a laparoscopic procedure.
- Histologic sampling of endometriotic lesions confirms the diagnosis.
- Endometriosis cannot be definitely diagnosed with ultrasound or hysterosalpingogram.
- Ultrasound imaging can detect endometriomas and other nodularity that may suggest endometriosis.
- Physical exam findings that support the diagnosis include tenderness on bimanual exam, nodularity along the uterosacral ligaments and/or posterior fornix, and a nonmobile or fixed uterus due to inflammation.

Management[1,2]

- The management of endometriosis is accomplished through a stepwise approach with careful consideration to the patient's desire for future fertility and risk factors/contraindications for use of particular pharmaceutical options
- NSAIDS
- Combination contraceptives or progestin-only contraceptives
- Gonadotropin-releasing hormone (GnRH) agonists or antagonists with 2.5 mg of norethindrone daily
  - Some clinicians will add conjugated estrogens 0.625 mg daily to prevent bone loss and help decrease vasomotor symptoms.
- Aromatase inhibitors
- Laparoscopy with endometriotic ablation and removal of endometriomas
- Definitive surgical management with hysterectomy

REFERENCES

1. Sarajari S, Muse KN, Fox MD, et al. Endometriosis. In: DeCherney AH, Nathan L, Laufer N, Roman AS, ed. *Current Diagnosis and Treatment: Obstetrics and Gynecology.* New York, NY: McGraw-Hill Medical; 2013:911–919.
2. Gambone JC. Endometriosis and adenomyosis. In: Hacker NF, Gambone JC, Hobel CJ, eds. *Hacker and Moore's Essentials of Obstetrics and Gynecology.* 6th ed. Philadelphia, PA: Saunders/Elsevier; 2016:314-321.

GALACTORRHEA

Etiology
- Galactorrhea, a benign milky discharge from the nipples, often occurs bilaterally and can be caused by hyperprolactinemia.
- Dopamine 2 antagonists, atypical antipsychotics (particularly first generation), methyldopa, verapamil, and opioids have all been implicated in galactorrhea.

Epidemiology
- Up to 90% of women with hyperprolactinemia will experience galactorrhea.[1]

Clinical Presentation
- Patients will present with painless milky discharge, usually bilaterally.
- Sanguineous and serosanguineous discharge; breast changes such as skin dimpling, retractions, erythema; and a mass can be ominous signs, requiring evaluation by a breast surgeon.
- The physical exam should assess for bitemporal vision changes that could indicate a prolactinoma, and thyroid palpation to evaluate for thyroid masses or goiter.
- Patients with significant galactorrhea and hyperprolactinemia often present with amenorrhea.

Diagnosis
- It is important to diagnose the underlying cause of the galactorrhea.
- Laboratory testing includes thyroid-stimulating hormone (TSH), beta human chorionic gonadotropin (beta-HCG), serum prolactin, and renal function.
- MRI of the pituitary, with and without contrast, may reveal a prolactinoma.
  - Measurement of the size of the pituitary mass is important because treatment decisions are dependent on the size.

Management[2]
- The management of galactorrhea depends on the underlying etiology.
- If the patient is taking a medication that is causing the symptoms, patients must be reassured that the medication is causing the side effect. If the galactorrhea is bothersome, consultation with the prescriber is warranted to address tapering or changing the medication.
- If the patient has a macroadenoma (a prolactinoma >1 cm) or a microadenoma (prolactinoma <1 cm), treatment with a dopamine agonist is appropriate.
- Cabergoline and bromocriptine are two commonly used dopamine agonists.

- Transsphenoid surgical resection by a neurosurgeon can be considered if the patient has a macroadenoma and fails medical treatment.
- Adenomas larger than 3 cm are also amenable to surgical resection.

REFERENCES

1. Colao A, Sarno AD, Cappabianca P, et al. Gender differences in the prevalence, clinical features and response to cabergoline in hyperprolactinemia. *Eur J Endocrinol.* 2003;148(3):325–331.
2. Lake MG, Krook LS, Cruz SV. Pituitary adenomas: an overview. *Am Fam Physician.* 2013;88(5):319-327. https://www.aafp.org/afp/2013/0901/p319.html

GENITOURINARY SYNDROME OF MENOPAUSE

Etiology[1]

- Formerly called *vulvovaginal atrophy* and *atrophic vaginitis*
- Due to the lack of estrogen in postmenopausal women
- The loss of estrogen results in decreased elasticity of the vagina, thinning of vaginal epithelium, decreased lubrication, and increased vaginal pH

Epidemiology[1]

- Up to 60% of postmenopausal patients will experience at least some of the symptoms of genitourinary syndrome of menopause (GUSM).

Clinical Presentation[1]

- Patients will present with a spectrum of symptoms, including vaginal and/or vulvar dryness and burning; decreased vaginal lubrication during sexual activity; dyspareunia; postcoital bleeding or spotting; dysorgasmia or anorgasmia; and urinary urgency, frequency, and recurrent or recent urinary tract infections (UTIs; Table 2.2).
- Postmenopausal women, women who take aromatase inhibitors for breast cancer, and premenopausal oophorectomized women who have not taken

TABLE 2.2 Summary of GUSM

Common Symptoms	Treatment Options
Vaginal and/or vulvar dryness and burning	Hyaluronic-based vaginal lubricants
Decreased vaginal lubrication during sexual activity	Vaginal estrogen (creams, tablets, rings)
Dyspareunia	Vaginal DHEA (prasterone)
Postcoital bleeding or spotting	Ospemifene (oral)
Dysorgasmia or anorgasmia	Vaginal laser therapy
Urinary urgency, frequency, and recurrent or recent UTIs	

DHEA, dehydroepiandrosterone; GUSM, genitourinary syndrome of menopause; UTI, urinary tract infection.

supplementary estrogen may present with the signs and symptoms of GUSM.
- GUSM negatively effects overall quality of life so patients should be screened at their regular visits and periodically as needed.

Diagnosis
- Diagnosis of GUSM can be accomplished by history.
- Physical examination may reveal decreased vaginal rugae and vaginal pallor.

Management[1,2]
- Localized treatment may include vaginal lubricants, vaginal estrogen, and intravaginal dehydroepiandrosterone (DHEA) suppository.
- Vaginal lubricants with hyaluronic acid can be as effective as topical estrogen for treating the GUSM.
- Intravaginal estrogens come in a variety of forms, including creams, tablets, and rings.
- Ospemifene is a selective estrogen modulator. It is an agonist on the endometrium so consider using a progestin to protect against hyperplasia.
- ACOG does not support the use of systemic estrogen in a patient with GUSM without vasomotor symptoms.
- Other options include laser therapy.

REFERENCES

1. Kim H-J, Kang S-Y, Chung Y-Jet al. The recent review of the genitourinary syndrome of menopause. *J Menopausal Med.* 2015;21(2):65–71. doi:10.6118/jmm.2015.21.2.65
2. Pitsouni E, Grigoriadis T, Falagas MEet al. Laser therapy for the genitourinary syndrome of menopause: a systematic review and meta-analysis. *Maturitas.* 2017;103:78–88. doi:10.1016/j.maturitas.2017.06.029

INFERTILITY

Etiology
- A couple can be considered infertile if no conception occurs after 12 months of attempting conception without the use of any contraception, in women younger than 35 years.
- In women older than 35 years, infertility can be diagnosed when the couple has tried to conceive for 6 months.
- Infertility can be categorized as primary or secondary.
- *Primary infertility* describes a woman who has never conceived, and *secondary infertility* indicates a woman has had a successful conception in the past.

Epidemiology[1]

- Approximately 12% of women will experience impaired fertility during the reproductive life span.
- Male factors are responsible for about 25% of infertility, followed by ovarian dysfunction and tubal pathology.
- In about 30% of infertile couples, no male or female pathology is found. This is referred to as *unexplained infertility* or *subfertility*.

Clinical Presentation

- Women will present with an inability to conceive after attempting conception.

Diagnosis

- A careful history and physical examination are imperative when evaluating a patient for infertility.
- Some of the essential elements include a menstrual history, gravida and para status, obstetric history if available, history of STIs, and presence of other endocrinopathies such as thyroid disorders.
- Physical examination should focus on ruling out pituitary disease, thyroid disease, structural abnormalities of the pelvis, and pathology of the reproductive tract.
- It is important to rule out a male factor etiology, so a semen analysis must be ordered.
- Initial laboratory testing of the woman includes a thyroid-stimulating hormone (TSH), day 3 follicle-stimulating hormone (FSH) and estradiol, and anti-Müllerian hormone test.
- Imaging studies include a hysterosalpingogram to assess tubal patency.
- Pelvic ultrasound and diagnostic laparoscopy with hysteroscopy can be performed in select patients.

Management

- All patients must be counseled on the importance of tobacco cessation, reducing caffeine intake, and other lifestyle interventions as appropriate.
- All women seeking pregnancy should take 400 mcg of folic acid every day to help prevent neural tube defects.
- Management depends on the underlying etiology.
- Medical therapies include ovulation inductors such as clomiphene citrate, aromatase inhibitors, and FSH.
- Surgical therapies may include myomectomy, neosalpingostomy, and fimbrioplasty if structural abnormalities are present.
- In vitro procedures generally take place with reproductive endocrinologists in specialty clinics.

CLINICAL PEARL: All women who present with infertility must have their partner's semen analyzed as part of the initial workup.

REFERENCE

1. National Center for Health Statistics. Infertility. https://www.cdc.gov/nchs/fastats/infertility.htm

LEIOMYOMA

Etiology

- Risk factors include Black race, early menarche, and nulliparity.
- Research suggests a genetic predisposition.
- Other risk factors that may be associated with the development of leiomyoma include obesity, low level of vitamin D, consumption of red meat, and beer intake.

Epidemiology[1]

- More common in Black women. Present during the reproductive years.
- Up to 80% of Black women and 70% of White women have leiomyoma on pelvic ultrasound, even when asymptomatic.

Clinical Presentation[2,3]

- Many women are asymptomatic.
- Symptoms may include heavy menses, pelvic pressure, pelvic pain, constipation, frequent urination, and infertility, depending on the location of the mass.
- Sometimes a uterine mass or an irregularly shaped uterus can be palpated on bimanual exam.
- A mobile irregular uterus is likely to be due to leiomyoma.

Diagnosis[2,3]

- Definitive diagnosis can be made with pelvic ultrasound.
- A hysteroscopy or saline-infused sonogram can identify lesions that extend into the uterine cavity.
- MRI is reserved for complicated leiomyomatous conditions.
- They are classified by their anatomical location
  - Subserosal, submucosal, intramural (Figure 2.2)

Management[2,3]

- The management depends on the location of the fibroid(s), desire for preserved fertility, and patient symptoms.
- Can be divided into four categories: expectant, medical, surgical, and interventional radiologic procedures.
  - Expectant
    - Appropriate for asymptomatic women and women who decline medical or surgical management.

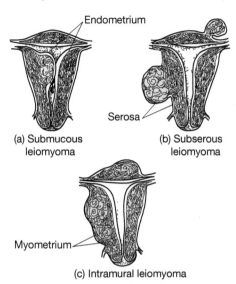

(a) Submucous
leiomyoma

(b) Subserous
leiomyoma

(c) Intramural leiomyoma

FIGURE 2.2 Appearance of uterine fibroids.

Source: Carcio HA, Secor RM. *Advanced health assessment of women: clinical skills and procedures.* 2nd ed. New York, NY: Springer Publishing Company; 2010.

- ○ Medical
  - ■ Combination contraceptives, progestin-only contraception (progestin-secreting intrauterine system [IUS]; progestin implants, injection, pills) to help with abnormal uterine bleeding
  - ■ Gonadotropin-releasing hormone (GnRH) agonists and antagonists
  - ■ Aromatase inhibitors
  - ■ Progesterone receptor modulators currently being studied
- ○ Surgical
  - ■ Myomectomy if anatomically amenable and patient desires future fertility
  - ■ Hysterectomy
  - ■ Endometrial ablation for heavy bleeding
- ○ Interventional radiologic procedures
  - ■ Uterine artery embolization

REFERENCES

1. Baird DD, Dunson DB, Hill MCet al. High cumulative incidence of uterine leiomyoma in black and white women: ultrasound evidence. *Am J Obstet Gynecol.* 2003;188(1):100–107. doi:10.1067/mob.2003.99
2. Parker WH, Gamboe JC. Benign conditions and congenital anomalies of the uterine corpus and cervix. In: Hacker NF, Gambone JC, Hobel CJ, eds. *Hacker and Moore's Essentials of Obstetrics and Gynecology.* 6th ed. Philadelphia, PA: Saunders/Elsevier; 2016:248–257.

3. American College of Obstetricians and Gynecologists. ACOG practice bulletin no. 96. Alternatives to hysterectomy in the management of leiomyomas. https://www.acog.org/Clinical-Guidance-and-Publications/Practice-Bulletins/Committee-on-Practice-Bulletins-Gynecology/Alternatives-to-Hysterectomy-in-the-Management-of-Leiomyomas. Published August 2008. Reaffirmed 2016.

MENOPAUSE

Etiology

- Menopause can occur naturally with a mean age of 51 years, surgically via oophorectomy, or prematurely, before age 40 years.
- Natural menopause is the permanent, unintentional cessation of menses 1 year after the last menstrual period.

Epidemiology

- All women who have not undergone oophorectomy will experience a natural decline in ovarian function followed by total ovarian follicle depletion, resulting in amenorrhea and other signs and symptoms of estrogen deficiency.
- Approximately one in 250 women will experience premature ovarian insufficiency by age 35 years, and one in 100 by age 40 years.[1]

Clinical Presentation

- Perimenopause can occur 4 to 5 years before the final last menstrual period and is marked by irregular menses, vasomotor symptoms, sleep disturbances, and mood changes.
- Women who are postmenopausal may often complain of vaginal dryness, urinary changes due to genitourinary atrophy, skin changes, cognitive changes, sleep disturbances, and sexual dysfunction.
- The *GUSM* is used to describe the dyspareunia, vaginal dryness and atrophy, and urinary symptoms that occur postmenopausally.

Diagnosis

- Diagnosis can be made by history.
- Menopause is signified by 1 year of amenorrhea not due to known pathology or intent to stop menses by any intervention in an appropriately aged woman.
- FSH will be elevated, with peak FSH occurring within the first few years after the final menstrual period.

- Perimenopause is marked by hormonal fluctuations, so FSH and estradiol levels are not diagnostic.
- Decreases in inhibin B and anti-Müellerian hormone are also present.

Management[2]

- During the perimenopause phase, it is important to try to maintain good bone health due to the loss of bone that occurs during this stage, so weight-bearing exercise should be encouraged.
- Postmenopausal women are at greater risk for heart disease, so proactive measures to maintain heart health are encouraged.
- Genitourinary symptoms can be treated with localized estrogen, hyaluronic-based vaginal moisturizers, DHEA preparations, or vaginal laser treatments (for more information, see "Genitourinary Syndrome of Menopause" in this chapter).
- Vasomotor symptoms and other somatic symptoms can be treated with systemic estrogen only if no contraindications exist and only after a careful risk–benefit discussion with the patient occurs.
- Women who desire systemic estrogen but still have a uterus must also use a progestin to protect against endometrial hyperplasia.
- The only other Food and Drug Administration (FDA)-approved treatment option for vasomotor symptoms includes paroxetine (a selective serotonin-reuptake inhibitor [SSRI]).
- Complementary therapies include yoga and acupuncture. Evidence is limited regarding their efficacy.
- ACOG recommends against the use of compounded hormones and other "natural" products, such as black cohosh, due to lack of FDA oversight.

> **CLINICAL PEARL:** Women who are going through the menopausal transition will commonly complain of forgetfulness. A mild cognitive decline is common among women, who typically return to baseline once through the transition. If there is significant concern about early-onset Alzheimer disease or frontotemporal dementia, a referral to a neuropsychiatrist is appropriate.

REFERENCES

1. Pellegrini VA. Ovarian insufficiency. In: Lucidi RS, ed. *Medscape.* https://emedicine.medscape.com/article/271046-overview#a7. Updated November 17, 2016.
2. American College of Obstetricians and Gynecologists. *Guidelines for Women's Health Care: A Resource Manual.* 4th ed. Washington, DC: Author; 2014. https://www.acog.org/Clinical-Guidance-and-Publications/Guidelines-for-Womens-Health-Care

OSTEOPOROSIS

Etiology[1]

- Osteoporosis is characterized by decrease in bone mass, distortion of bone microarchitecture, and an overall decline in the quality of bone.
- Several factors increase a woman's risk for developing osteoporosis, including aging, menopause, aromatase inhibitor use for breast cancer, chronic corticosteroid use, tobacco use, anorexia nervosa, chronic medroxyrogesterone use without estrogen, sedentarism, and nutritional deficiencies, particularly vitamin D and calcium.
- Secondary causes of osteoporosis can be caused by thyroid dysfunction, celiac disease, and parathyroid dysfunction.
- Disorders that are associated with the development of osteoporosis include rheumatoid arthritis, lupus, Cushing syndrome, adrenal insufficiency, gastric bypass, inflammatory bowel disease, cystic fibrosis, alcoholism, and seizure disorders.
- Other pharmaceuticals that can cause osteoporosis include antiseizure medications, lithium, and some antineoplastics.

Epidemiology

- Women are 5 times as likely as men to develop osteoporosis.[1]
- It is expected that by the year 2020, 12.3 million people 50 years and older will be diagnosed with osteoporosis in the United States.[2]
- More than half of women age 80 years and older who sustain a hip fracture will be unable to walk without assistance 1 year post fracture.[3]
- Up to 6% of women age 80 years and older will die during hospitalization for a hip fracture.[2]

Clinical Presentation

- The vast majority of women will be asymptomatic.
- Sometimes a patient will present with a recent long bone fracture and subsequent testing reveals osteoporosis.

Diagnosis

- The gold standard for diagnosing osteoporosis is the dual-energy x-ray absorptiometry, or DEXA, of the hip and lumbar spine.
- The femoral neck, total hip, and lumbar spine bone mineral density are measured and compared with the mean bone mineral density of young, otherwise healthy women. This is called the *T-score* (Table 2.3).
  - A T-score less than or equal to −2.5 for any of the three sites is diagnostic for osteoporosis
- Bone turnover biomarkers should not be used to diagnose osteoporosis.

TABLE **2.3** Diagnosis of Osteoporosis

Categorization	T-Score
Normal bone mineral density	≥ -1.0
Low bone mass (formerly referred to as *osteopenia*)	Between -1.0 and -2.5
Osteoporosis	≤ -2.5

- The Z-score compares the patient's bone mineral density to that of an average in women of her age. Knowing their Z-score could be helpful to younger women.
- It may be appropriate to check for secondary causes of osteoporosis in young women without apparent risk factors.
- Screening guidelines for osteoporosis vary slightly by organization:
  - The National Osteoporosis Foundation (NOF) recommends a DEXA scan in women 65 years and older, menopausal with risk factors, and in postmenopausal women younger than 65 years with risk factors.[4]
  - The United States Preventive Services Taskforce (USPSTF)[5] recommends the following as Grade B:
    - Women 65 years and older should have their bone density evaluated.
    - Postmenopausal women who are younger than 65 years with risk factors for osteoporosis should undergo bone density screening.
  - The NOF and USPSTF both state that there is insufficient evidence to recommend a duration of time between screenings.
- One study[6] recommended that women older than 65 years with normal bone mineral density undergo rescreening every 15 years; if the T-score is between -1.5 and -1.99, women should undergo rescreening every 5 years; and women with a T-score between -2.0 and -2.49 should undergo rescreening annually.
- Fracture risk assessment tool (FRAX) screening should occur annually in all women older than 65 years.

Management[1]

- The World Health Organization helped to develop the FRAX. The FRAX score helps to stratify patients by their risk of sustaining an osteoporotic fracture within the next 10 years. See www.sheffield.ac.uk/FRAX/ for more information.
- Management can be divided into pharmacologic and lifestyle interventions (Table 2.4).
- Bisphosphonates inhibit osteoclast resorption of bone and as such are called *antiresorptive medications*.
  - Bisphosphonates include risedronate, alendronate, ibandronate, and zoledronate.
  - Alendronate and zoledronate significantly reduce hip fractures, but all bisphosphonates reduce vertebral fractures.

TABLE 2.4 Summary of Interventions for Osteoporosis Prevention and Treatment

Pharmacologic	Lifestyle
Bisphosphonates	Tobacco and alcohol cessation
SERM (raloxifene)	Increase exercise (weight-bearing, muscle-strengthening)
Calcitonin salmon	Daily calcium and vitamin D
Recombinant human parathyroid hormone	Fall risk education
RANK ligand inhibitor	

RANK, receptor activator of nuclear factor; SERM, selective estrogen receptor modulator.

- ○ Zolendronate is an intravenous formulation, whereas the others are orally administered. Patients must be screened for renal disease prior to administering zolendronate.
- ○ Bisphosphonates are associated with gastrointestinal (GI) upset, esophageal cancer, and osteonecrosis of the jaw.
- Raloxifene is a selective estrogen receptor modulator. It is indicated for the prevention of osteoporosis in women at risk and for the treatment of osteoporosis.
- ○ Contraindications to raloxifene include a history of thromboembolic events and pregnancy.
- ○ It is not indicated for premenopausal women.
- Calcitonin-salmon intranasal preparations are indicated for osteoporosis by the FDA, but have less efficacy than other treatment options.
- ○ Patients with an existing fracture, particularly of the vertebral column, may achieve mild analgesia when using intranasal calcitonin salmon.
- Teriparatide, recombinant human parathyroid hormone, is indicated for patients with an elevated fracture risk. It is a daily subcutaneous injection.
- ○ Side effects include angioedema and anaphylaxis.
- ○ There is a black-box warning for osteosarcoma.
- Denosumab, a receptor activator of NF-κB (RANK) ligand inhibitor, is indicated for the treatment of osteoporosis in high-risk patients by the FDA.
- ○ Denosumab is a subcutaneous injection administered by a healthcare provider every 6 months. Hypocalcemia is a contraindication, so patients must have a serum calcium level checked prior to administration.
- Lifestyle interventions include weight-bearing exercises, muscle-strengthening exercises, tobacco and alcohol cessation, and daily calcium and vitamin D intake.
- ○ Women 51 to 70 years should have a minimum daily intake of 1,200 mg of calcium and 600 IU of vitamin D.
- ○ Women 71 years and older should have a minimum daily intake of 1,200 mg of calcium and 800 IU of vitamin D.

- All patients with osteoporosis should have a fall evaluation and be educated on fall-prevention measures.
  - ○ Fall-prevention measures include the use of nonskid rugs; adequate and accessible lighting in all rooms; nightlights; removal of any items that can impede walking, including cords and other items that can cause a fall; safety handles and bars in the bathroom, both by the toilet and in the shower/bath; and avoidance of placing items in high spaces that require women to use stepstools or ladders to reach them.

References

1. American College of Obstetricians and Gynecologists. ACOG Practice Bulletin no. 129. Osteoporosis. *Obstet Gynecol*. 2012, 120(3):718–734. doi:10.1097/AOG.0b013e31826dc45d

2. Wright NC, Looker AC, Saag KG, et al. The recent prevalence of osteoporosis and low bone mass in the United States based on bone mineral density at the femoral neck or lumbar spine. *J Bone Miner Res*. 2014;29(11):2520-2526. doi:10.1002/jbmr.2269

3. Boonen S, Autier P, Barette M, et al. Functional outcome and quality of life following hip fracture in elderly women: a prospective controlled study. *Osteoporos Int*. 2004;15:87-94. doi:10.1007/s00198-003-1515-z

4. National Osteoporosis Foundation. Bone density exam/testing. https://www.nof.org/patients/diagnosis-information/bone-density-examtesting

5. United States Preventive Services Taskforce. Final recommendation statement. Osteoporosis to prevent fractures: screening. https://www.uspreventiveservicestaskforce.org/Page/Document/RecommendationStatementFinal/osteoporosis-screening1

6. Gourlay ML, Fine JP, Preisser JS, et al. Bone-density testing interval and transition to osteoporosis in older women. Study of osteoporotic fractures research group. *N Engl J Med*. 2012;366:225-233. doi:10.1056/NEJMoa1107142

Ovarian Cancer

Etiology[1,2]

- Ninety-five percent of ovarian carcinomas are epithelial.
- Serous ovarian carcinoma, a subtype of epithelial cancer, is related fallopian tube and peritoneal cancer, and comprises about 75% of epithelial carcinomas.
- Other histological subtypes of epithelial ovarian cancer are clear cell, endometrioid, and mucinous.
- Nonepithelial etiologies include germ cell and sex-cord stromal ovarian carcinomas.
- Risk factors for the development of ovarian cancer include *BRCA* 1 or 2 mutation, Lynch syndrome (hereditary nonpolyposis colorectal cancer [HNPCC]), late age at menopause (>52 years), nulliparity, endometriosis, and cigarette smoking.

- Protective factors include oral contraceptive use, multiparity, salpingo-oopherectomy, tubal ligation, breastfeeding, and hysterectomy.

Epidemiology[1,2,3]

- Ovarian cancer is the second most common gynecologic malignancy, but is the leading cause of death among gynecologic malignancies.
- Approximately 1.3% of women in the United States will be diagnosed with ovarian cancer at some point in their lives.
- Women with *BRCA1* mutations have an estimated lifetime risk of developing ovarian cancer of almost 50%, and *BRCA2* of almost 25%.
- Women with Lynch syndrome (HNPCC) have a lifetime risk of 14%.
- Epithelial ovarian cancer is commonly diagnosed at an advanced stage, with 65% of women diagnosed at stage III or stage IV, when the cure rate is only 18%,

Clinical Presentation[3,4]

- Some women will present with a condition due to advanced ovarian cancer such as ascites, pleural effusion, and bowel obstruction.
- Others will present with vague complaints such as pelvic pain or pressure, bloating, early satiety.
- Sometimes an ovarian cancer will be an incidental finding on pelvic ultrasound or in the workup of a patient with pelvic complaints.

Diagnosis[3,4]

- Diagnosis is made histologically through surgery.
- However, a thorough preoperative evaluation is undertaken to assess the possibility of metastatic disease and the need for presurgical chemotherapy.
- Presurgical imaging is done with pelvic and abdominal CT unless the patient has a contraindication to CT dye, in which case an MRI can be completed.
- A chest x-ray is also performed to assess for presence of pleural effusions, metastases, and hilar lymphadenopathy.
- Laboratory testing includes CA-125.
  - CA-125 should not be used as a screening test in asymptomatic women.
- There are several commercially available ovarian cancer panels that can be used.
  - These include CA-125 but may also test for beta 2 microglobulin, apolipoprotein A1, FSH, transferrin, and transthyretin.
- The Risk of Malignancy Algorithm (ROMA) uses human epididymis secretory protein 4 (HE4) and CA-125 combined with a computer regression algorithm that provides a risk-of-malignancy score based on a woman's menopausal status.
- Ovarian cancer is staged from IA to IV using the FIGO/TNM system.[5]
- Each stage is further divided, depending on location, size of lymph nodes, and location of metastases:
  - Stage I: Tumor confined to an ovary

○ Stage II: Tumor involves one or both ovaries with pelvic extension below the pelvic brim, or peritoneal cancer
○ Stage III: Tumor involves one or both ovaries with peritoneal spread outside the pelvis and/or metastasis to retroperitoneal lymph nodes
○ Stage IV: Distant metastases, excluding peritoneal metastases

Management[3,4]

- Management of ovarian cancer is largely dependent upon stage and histology.
- Hysterectomy and BSO with pelvic and para-aortic lymph node dissection, pelvic washing cytology, and omenectomy are performed.
- If metastatic disease is present, bowel resection and partial hepatic resection may be performed.
- Platinum-based chemotherapy is used for either adjuvant or neoadjuvant options and includes carboplatin and cisplatin.

REFERENCES

1. National Cancer Institute Cancer stat facts: ovarian cancer. https://seer.cancer.gov/statfacts/html/ovary.html
2. Barrow E, Robinson L, Alduaij W, et al. Cumulative lifetime incidence of extra-colonic cancers in Lynch syndrome: a report of 121 families with proven mutations. *Clin Genet.* 2009;75(2):141–149. doi:10.1111/j.1399-0004.2008.01125.x
3. American College of Obstetricians and Gynecologists. ACOG committee opinion no. 716: the role of the obstetrician-gynecologist in the early detection of epithelial ovarian cancer in women at average risk. https://www.acog.org/Clinical-Guidance-and-Publications/Committee-Opinions/Committee-on-Gynecologic-Practice/The-Role-of-the-Obstetrician-Gynecologist-in-the-Early-Detection-of-Epithelial-Ovarian-Cancer-in. Published September 2017.
4. Levy G, Purcell K. Premalignant and malignant disorders of the ovaries and oviducts. In: DeCherney AH, Nathan L, Laufer N, Roman AS, ed. *Current Diagnosis and Treatment: Obstetrics and Gynecology.* New York, NY: McGraw-Hill Medical; 2013:848–858.
5. Society for Gynecologic Oncology. FIGO ovarian cancer staging. https://www.sgo.org/wp-content/uploads/2012/09/FIGO-Ovarian-Cancer-Staging_1.10.14.pdf

OVARIAN CYSTS

Etiology

- Physiologic (corpus luteal or follicular) or polycystic ovaries
- Ovarian cysts are hormonally driven, thus occurring primarily in reproductive-aged women, but can occur premenarche or postmenopause

Epidemiology[1]

- About 70% of ovarian masses are benign ovarian cysts.

Clinical Presentation[1,2]

- May be asymptomatic and found incidentally on ultrasound.
- The patient may complain of pelvic pain and fullness.
- If a cyst ruptures, it may cause acute pain and hemoperitoneum.
- If ovarian torsion occurs, there may be considerable pain.

Diagnosis[1,2]

- Normal ovulatory cysts are smaller than 3 cm.
- Larger cysts may be palpable on bimanual exam.
- Definitive diagnosis is accomplished via pelvic ultrasound.
- A simple, unilocular, hypo- or anechoic, thin-walled cyst is the classic description of a benign follicular ovarian cyst.
- A corpus luteal cyst can have thick vascular walls and internal debris.
- Follicular and corpus luteal cysts are usually between 3 and 5 cm but can be much larger when they fail to be reabsorbed.

Management[1,2]

- All patients should be evaluated for their risk factors for ovarian cancer (see "Ovarian Cancer").
- Cystic or mixed lesions with multiloculations, solid areas, and ascites must be ruled out as malignant.
- Management of smaller cysts in younger women who are asymptomatic or mildly symptomatic can often be expectant.
- A repeat ultrasound performed 6 weeks after the initial scan may reveal regression, growth, or other changes.
  - A repeat scan can also be done at 3 months to evaluate change.
- Cysts larger than 10 cm are typically removed via laparoscopy, and any ovarian mass that has characteristics of neoplasm in a patient with risk factors for ovarian cancer, including an elevated CA-125, should be removed surgically.
- Please note that CA-125 is not recommended for screening an asymptomatic patient for ovarian cancer.

> **Clinical Pearl:** The size of the cyst does not correlate with the level of pain the patient may experience.

References

1. Parker WH, Gmbone JC. Congenital anomalies and benign conditions of the ovaries and fallopian tubes. In: Hacker NF, Gambone JC, Hobel CJ, eds. *Hacker and Moore's Essentials of Obstetrics and Gynecology.* 6th ed. Philadelphia, PA: Saunders/Elsevier; 2016:248–257.
2. American College of Obstetricians and Gynecologists. ACOG practice bulletin no 174: evaluation and management of adnexal masses. https://www.acog.org/Clinical-Guidance-and-Publications/Practice-Bulletins/Committee-on-Practice-Bulletins-Gynecology/Evaluation-and-Management-of-Adnexal-Masses. Published November 2016.

PELVIC INFLAMMATORY DISEASE

Etiology
- PID is usually caused by chlamydia or gonorrhea, but there are cases in which *Mycoplasma hominis* has been identified as well.
  - Occasionally, other organisms will be identified, including *Gardnerella vaginalis, Haemophilus influenzae*, and *Streptococcus agalactiae*.

Epidemiology
- According to the CDC, the self-reported lifetime prevalence is 4.4%, or 2.5 million women have been diagnosed with PID.[1]

Clinical Presentation
- Signs and symptoms can vary, depending on the severity of infection.
- Most women will complain of pelvic pain and/or lower abdominal pain.
- Some women will present with a vaginal discharge that is purulent.
- Fever may be present but is not required to diagnose PID.

Diagnosis
- The classic triad of uterine tenderness, cervical motion tenderness, and adnexal tenderness in a sexually active woman with lower abdominal or pelvic pain is usually indicative of PID.
- Although laparoscopy can confirm the diagnosis, it is not necessary.
- Microscopy of vaginal discharge usually reveals white blood cells.
- A CBC may reveal an elevated white blood cell count with a left shift.
- Specimens from the endocervix may show the causative organisms, but some women with PID will have negative endocervical testing.
- Thus, the diagnosis of PID is usually made by history and physical examination when there is an index of suspicion for PID.
- Patients who present with fever, an elevated white count and a left shift, and an adnexal mass should be evaluated for a possible tubo-ovarian abscess.

Management
- Management options depend on whether or not the patient is being treated as an outpatient or an inpatient and if the patient is pregnant as doxycycline should not be used in pregnancy (Table 2.5).
- **Outpatient treatment**[2,3]
  - Preferred antimicrobial option: Ceftriaxone 250 mg intramuscularly plus doxycycline 100 mg orally twice a day for 14 days; can consider metronidazole 500 mg orally twice a day for 14 days if you suspect an anaerobic etiology.
  - Alternate option: Cefoxitin 2 g intramuscularly plus probenecid 1 g orally in a single dose, plus doxycycline 100 mg orally twice a day for 14

TABLE 2.5 Overview of the Management of PID

Outpatient Treatment	Inpatient Treatment
CDC preferred option: Ceftriaxone 250 mg intramuscularly	CDC preferred option: Cefotetan 2 g intravenously
PLUS Doxycycline 100 mg orally twice a day for 14 days Can consider metronidazole 500 mg orally twice a day for 14 days if suspicious of an anaerobic etiology	OR Cefoxitin 2 g intravenously every 6 hours PLUS Doxycycline 100 mg orally or intravenously every 12 hours
CDC alternate option: Cefoxitin 2 g intramuscularly PLUS Probenecid 1 g orally in a single dose PLUS Doxycycline 100 mg orally twice a day for 14 days Can consider metronidazole 500 mg orally twice a day for 14 days if suspicious of an anaerobic etiology	CDC alternative option: Clindamycin 900 mg intravenously every 8 hours PLUS Gentamicin 2 mg/kg loading dose intravenously followed by 1.5 mg/kg maintenance dose every 8 hours (can also use daily dosing of gentamicin 3–5 mg/kg)

CDC, Centers for Disease Control and Prevention; PID, pelvic inflammatory disease.

days; can consider metronidazole 500 mg orally twice a day for 14 days if you suspect an anaerobic etiology.

- **Inpatient treatment**[2–4]
  - Inpatient treatment should be considered for any woman with the following:
    - Pelvic abscess
    - Pregnancy
    - Immunodeficiency
    - Failure to show clinical improvement after 72 hours of outpatient treatment
    - Inability to tolerate oral medications
    - Concern for compliance with outpatient regimen
  - Preferred antimicrobial option: Cefotetan 2 g intravenously or cefoxitin 2 g intravenously every 6 hours plus doxycycline 100 mg orally or intravenously every 12 hours
  - Alternative option: Clindamycin 900 mg intravenously every 8 hours plus gentamicin 2 mg/kg loading dose intravenously followed by 1.5 mg/kg maintenance dose every 8 hours (can also use daily dosing of gentamicin 3 to 5 mg/kg)

References

1. Kreisel K, Torrone E, Bernstein K, et al. Prevalence of pelvic inflammatory disease in sexually experienced women of reproductive age — United States, 2013–2014. *Morb Mortal Wkly Rep*. 2017;66(3):80–83. doi:10.15585/mmwr.mm6603a3

2. Mackay G. Sexually transmitted diseases and pelvic infections. In: DeCherney AH, Nathan L, Laufer N, Roman AS, ed. *Current Diagnosis and Treatment: Obstetrics and Gynecology*. New York, NY: McGraw-Hill Medical; 2013:701–731.

3. Tough DeSapri KA. Pelvic inflammatory disease. In: Karjane NW, ed. *Medscape*. https://emedicine.medscape.com/article/256448-overview. Updated May 3, 2019.

4. Centers for Disease Control and Prevention. 2015 sexually transmitted diseases treatment guidelines: pelvic inflammatory disease. https://www.cdc.gov/std/tg2015/pid.htm

Pelvic Organ Prolapse: Cystocele, Rectocele, and Uterine Prolapse

Etiology[1]

- Pelvic organ prolapse occurs when pelvic floor laxity is present, allowing the anterior vaginal wall, posterior vaginal wall, apex (posthysterectomy), and/or uterus to descend.
- Risk factors for the development of pelvic organ prolapse include a prior history of vaginal delivery, advancing age, obesity, prior pregnancy, connective tissue disease, estrogen deficiency, and chronic constipation.

Epidemiology

- Approximately 3% of women will complain of pelvic organ prolapse, but as many as 50% of women will have evidence of some prolapse on physical exam.

Clinical Presentation

- Most women are asymptomatic, particularly in early stages.
- Symptoms, if present, include a vaginal bulge, pelvic pressure, urinary frequency or incontinence, constipation, and sexual dysfunction.
- Diagnosis
  - Diagnosis is made by physical examination.
  - ACOG recommends using the Pelvic Organ Prolapse Quantification (POP-Q) examination measurements to more adequately quantify the presence of prolapse.
  - Pelvic organ prolapse is graded from 0 to IV(Figure 2.3).
    - Stage 0: No prolapse present
    - Stage I: Most distal prolapse is greater than1 cm above the introitus

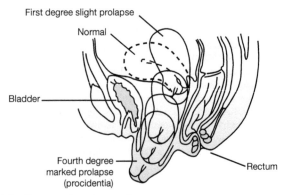

FIGURE 2.3 Degree of uterine prolapse.
Source: Secor RM, Fantasia HC. *Fast Facts About the Gynecologic Exam.* 2nd ed. New York, NY: Springer Publishing Company; 2018:33.

- Stage II: Most distal prolapse is between 1 cm above or below the introitus
- Stage III: Most distal prolapse is greater than 1 cm below the introitus but no more than 2 cm less than the total vaginal length
- Stage IV: Most distal prolapse is at least 2 cm below the introitus; this is called *procidentia*

Management

- Management depends on the grade of prolapse, the symptoms present, and patient preference.
- Lifestyle modifications are appropriate for lower grade prolapse, particularly when symptomatic. For example, women with chronic constipation should be offered patient education on increasing fiber and water intake.
- Pelvic-muscle strengthening can prevent the worsening of early prolapse.
- Referral to a physical therapist with training in pelvic floor muscle strengthening is often indicated.
- Various pessaries are available depending on the extent and location of prolapse.
- Ring pessaries are effective in most patients with grade II prolapse, whereas patients with grade IV usually require a Gellhorn pessary.
- Surgery is reserved for women who fail conservative management.
- Various surgical interventions are available and depend on the extent of prolapse and the presence or absence of more than one vaginal wall prolapse.

REFERENCE

1. American College of Obstetricians ad Gynecologists. Practice bulletin no. 185. Pelvic organ prolapse. https://www.acog.org/Clinical-Guidance-and-Publications/Practice-Bulletins/Committee-on-Practice-Bulletins-Gynecology/Pelvic-Organ-Prolapse. Published November 2017.

POLYCYSTIC OVARIAN SYNDROME

Etiology

- There is evidence that an abnormality of cytochrome P450c17 17-hydroxylase may be responsible for androgen biosynthesis that results in the hyperandrogenism seen in patients with polycystic ovarian syndrome (PCOS).[1]
- Patients with PCOS also manifest insulin resistance and ovulatory dysfunction.
- Some patients will have multiple cysts on their ovaries.
- Obesity will worsen symptoms but is not a cause of PCOS.

Epidemiology[1]

- There are various diagnostic criteria used for PCOS, so true incidence is difficult to assess.
- Incidence may be around 7%.[1]

Clinical Presentation

- Most women with PCOS will present with menstrual irregularities.
- Patients may be oligomenorrheic or amenorrheic.
- Patients may have type 2 diabetes or evidence of insulin resistance.
- Often, patients with PCOS will present with infertility.
- Some patients with PCOS may be hypertensive and have dyslipidemia.
- Other phenotypic evidence of PCOS includes hirsutism, androgenic alopecia, acanthosis nigricans, and central adiposity.

Diagnosis

- Diagnostic criteria vary by professional organization.
- Patients must have evidence of oligo- or amenorrhea and hyperandrogenism.
- Polycystic ovaries visualized on ultrasound are not a requirement for diagnosis.
- Laboratory diagnostics include the following:
  - ○ Evidence of hyperandrogenism as manifested by low sex hormone binding globulin and elevated total testosterone

○ Exclusion of alternative causes of hyperandrogenism and menstrual irregularities, when applicable, such as Cushing syndrome, thyroid dysfunction, 21-hydroxylase deficiency, and hyperprolactinemia.

○ Evidence of metabolic syndrome, including dyslipidemia and impaired glucose tolerance or diabetes.

Management[1]

- The goal of treatment is to mitigate the long-term cardiovascular and metabolic effects of PCOS and to protect the endometrium from hyperplasia and subsequent cancer (Table 2.6).
- Management should include patient education on lifestyle changes, such as increased exercise, to help patients lose weight if they are obese.
- Patients should be monitored regularly for hypertension, dyslipidemia, and insulin resistance/diabetes.
- Weight loss may help to reestablish menses.
  - ○ A 5% loss in total body weight has been shown to improve metabolic parameters and result in spontaneous menses.[1]
  - ○ Patients need to be counseled that conception can occur during this time.
- Metformin has been shown to increase insulin sensitivity.
- If patients do not wish to conceive, combined hormonal contraceptives or progestin-only contraceptives may be used in the absence of contraindications.
- Spironolactone is an aldosterone and androgen antagonist. It has been used to mitigate the phenotypical presentation of PCOS, including hirsutism. It may also help to reestablish menses.
  - ○ Spironolactone is dosed at 25 mg twice daily with gradual titration up to 100 mg twice daily.

TABLE 2.6 Overview of PCOS Treatment Options

Fertility Status	Treatment Options
Not desiring conception	Weight loss if overweight/obese
	Combined contraception
	Episodic progestin or progesterone × 10 days to induce withdrawal bleed
	Metformin to increase insulin sensitivity
	Spironolactone for hirsutism
	Finasteride for androgenic alopecia
	Eflornithine hydrochloride cream 13.9% for hirsutism
	Management of dyslipidemia and cardiovascular sequelae as appropriate
Desiring conception	Weight loss if overweight/obese
	Folic acid 400 mcg/d
	Progestin or progesterone × 10 days to induce withdrawal bleed
	Ovulation induction with clomiphene citrate or letrozole

PCOS, polycystic ovarian syndrome.

- ○ Side effects of spironolactone include hypotension and hyperkalemia.
- ○ Spironolactone should never be used in pregnancy or in women who wish to conceive.
- ○ Finasteride is a 5-alpha reductase inhibitor. It can be used for androgenic alopecia.
  - ▪ Finasteride is dosed at 1 mg each day.
  - ▪ Finasteride is teratogenic to male fetuses and should never be used in pregnancy or in women who wish to conceive.
- Eflornithine hydrochloride cream 13.9%, a topical preparation, is approved by the FDA for hirsutism in women.
- In patients who wish to conceive, ovulation induction is indicated.
- Patients who wish to conceive must be advised to begin folic acid supplementation right away.
- Patients who are amenorrheic may be given progesterone for 10 days to induce a withdrawal bleed as both drugs used to induce ovulation are timed according to day of menses.
- Clomiphene citrate and letrozole are used to induce ovulation in patients with PCOS.
  - ○ Clomiphene citrate is an estrogen-receptor antagonist. Its use forces increased gonadotropic secretion from the pituitary gland.
  - ○ The dosage of clomiphene citrate is 50 mg daily for 5 days.
  - ○ Letrozole is an aromatase inhibitor. Letrozole also increases pituitary gonadotropin secretion.
  - ○ The dosage of letrozole is 2.5 mg daily for 5 days.
  - ○ Of note, recent studies have shown that letrozole is more effective at inducing ovulation and subsequent live births than clomiphene citrate, particularly in women with PCOS.[1]
  - ○ Both clomiphene citrate and letrozole can result in multiple gestations.

REFERENCE

1. Lucidi RS. Polycystic ovarian syndrome. In: Lucidi RS, ed. *Medscape*. https://emedicine.medscape.com/article/256806-overview. Updated February 28, 2018.

PREMENSTRUAL SYNDROME/PREMENSTRUAL DYSPHORIC DISORDER

Etiology

- The etiology of premenstrual syndrome (PMS)/premenstrual dysphoric disorder (PMDD) is poorly understood, but there is consensus that the pathophysiology underlying PMS/PMDD is an abnormal response to ovarian steroids.

- The affective complaints are likely associated with changes in serotonergic receptors during the menstrual cycle.[1]

Epidemiology

- Up to 80% of women will experience one or more premenstrual symptom, but only about 8% of patients fit the *Diagnostic and Statistical Manual of Mental Disorders*, Fifth Edition (*DSM-5*) diagnostic criteria for PMDD.[2]

Clinical Presentation

- The presentation of PMS/PMDD can be categorized into affective and somatic complaints (Table 2.7).
- Affective complaints include mood swings, anxiety, increased irritability, dysthymic mood, and appetite changes.
- Physical complaints include bloating, fatigue, breast tenderness, headaches, and somnolence.
- *DSM-5* requires documentation that symptoms negatively affect a patient's quality of life.

Diagnosis[3]

- Diagnosis can be made by a careful history and physical examination.
- Patients who experience severe affective symptoms are more likely to have PMDD, particularly if the symptoms negatively affect the quality of life.
- Affective symptoms include depression, irritability, social withdrawal, anxiety, confusion, and anger outbursts.
- Somatic symptoms include breast tenderness, bloating, headache, myalgias/arthralgias, weight gain, and edema.
- One somatic symptom that occurs during the luteal phase and resolves after menstruation is likely PMS.
- ACOG has defined *PMS* as a condition in which a woman experiences at least one affective symptom and one somatic symptom that cause dysfunction in social, academic, or work performance.

TABLE 2.7 PMS/PMDD Symptoms

Affective Symptoms	Somatic Symptoms
Depression	Breast tenderness
Irritability	Bloating
Social withdrawal	Headache
Anxiety	Myalgias
Confusion	Arthralgias
Angry outbursts	Weight gain
	Edema

PMS, premenstrual syndrome; PMDD, premenstrual dysphoric disorder.

- Five or more symptoms that resolve within a week of onset menses, that includes an affective symptom, for at least three consecutive menstrual cycles, is likely PMDD.

Management

- SSRIs are indicated for PMS/PMDD.
- Combination contraception may be helpful for some women.
- In addition, 500 mg of calcium taken twice daily may relieve some symptoms.

REFERENCES

1. Halbreich U. The etiology, biology, and evolving pathology of premenstrual syndromes. *Psychoneuroendocrinology*. 2003;28(suppl 3):55–99. doi:10.1016/S0306 -4530(03)00097-0
2. Wittchen H-U, Becker E, Lieb R, Krause P. Prevalence, incidence and stability of premenstrual dysphoric disorder in the community. *Psychol Med*. 2002;32(1):119– 132. doi:10.1017/S0033291701004925
3. American College of Obstetricians and Gynecologists. *Guidelines for Women's Health Care: A Resource Manual*. 4th ed. Washington, DC: American College of Obstetricians and Gynecologists; 2014. https://www.acog.org/Clinical-Guidance -and-Publications/Guidelines-for-Womens-Health-Care

SEXUAL DYSFUNCTION

Etiology[1]

- The etiology of female sexual dysfunction can be multifactorial.
- Women who are postmenopausal and have GUSM are more likely to develop a sexual disorder.
- Medication use can decrease sexual desire in women.
  - ○ SSRIs are known to cause sexual dysfunction.
- Women who are depressed are more likely to develop a sexual disorder.
- Traumatic events may cause women to develop a sexual disorder.
- Women with anorgasmia often have a history of abuse or trauma.
- Women who experience pain with sexual intercourse due to vestibulitis, vulvodynia, interstitial cystitis, pelvic congestion syndrome, endometriosis, and adenomyosis may develop a sexual disorder.
- For a review of pelvic pain etiology, see the section "Pelvic Pain" in Chapter 1, Common Presentations in OB/GYN.

Epidemiology[1]

- An estimated 13% of women experience hypoactive sexual desire disorder.
- Approximately 5% of women will have a sexual arousal disorder.

- The actual incidence is probably higher than reported in the literature due to lack of reporting.

Clinical Presentation

- Patients may present with loss of libido or sexual desire, sexual arousal impairment, difficulty achieving or inability to achieve orgasm, and dyspareunia.
- Symptoms result in decreased quality of life.

Diagnosis[2]

- The *DSM-5* lists three types of female sexual dysfunction:
  - Sexual interest/arousal disorder encompasses hypoactive desire dysfunction and arousal dysfunction, previously listed as separate entities in earlier iterations of the *DSM*.
  - Dyspareunia and vaginismus are referred to as *genitopelvic pain/penetration disorder*
  - Female orgasmic disorder is unchanged in *DSM-5*.
- *DSM-5* requires symptoms be present for at least 6 months.

Management[1,3]

- Management depends on the patient's medical, surgical, and psychiatric history; medication use; and menopausal status.
- Postmenopausal women with GUSM may benefit from topical estrogens, DHEA inserts, and hyaluronic acid–based lubricants.
- The FDA has approved two oral drugs for hypoactive sexual disorder in premenopausal women, flibanserin and bremelanotide.
- Patients who are taking medications known to decrease libido and that can cause sexual dysfunction may require reconsideration of the medication with the prescriber.
- The FDA has approved a clitoral suction device that may help women with orgasm dysfunction and decreased arousal.
  - The device is currently available by prescription.[3]
- Transdermal testosterone formulations may improve symptoms of sexual dysfunction but are not considered safe if used for more than 6 months.
- Referral to a therapist who is knowledgeable about sexual disorders can be beneficial.

REFERENCES

1. American College of Obstetricians and Gynecologists. ACOG practice bulletin no. 213. Female sexual dysfunction. https://www.acog.org/Clinical-Guidance-and-Publications/Practice-Bulletins/Committee-on-Practice-Bulletins-Gynecology/Female-Sexual-Dysfunction. Accessed July 28, 2018. Published June 25, 2019.
2. Ishak WW, Tobia G. DSM 5 changes in diagnostic criteria of sexual dysfunctions. *Reprod Sys Sex Disord*. 2013;2:122. doi:10.4172/2161-038X.1000122
3. Nugyn. Eros therapy device. http://eros-therapy.com/products-page/eros-products/eros-therapy-device

Tubo-Ovarian Abscess

Etiology[1]
- Tubo-ovarian abscesses are infectious adnexal masses resulting from PID.
- The most common organisms are *Bacteroides* and *Escherichia coli* even though gonorrhea and chlamydia are associated with PID.

Epidemiology[1]
- Tubo-ovarian abscesses almost always occur in reproductive-aged patients.
- The CDC reports an incidence of tubo-ovarian abscess of about 2.3% in patients with PID.

Clinical Presentation[1]
- The presentation of a tubo-ovarian abscess can be variable, but the typical presentation includes abdominal and/or pelvic pain, an adnexal mass on bimanual examination, fever, and leukocytosis.
- Other symptoms may include nausea, chills, vaginal discharge, and irregular vaginal bleeding.
- Patients may also present with peritonitis.
- A patient with a ruptured tubo-ovarian abscess may present in sepsis.

Diagnosis[1]
- Patients with suspicion for PID should have a speculum and bimanual exam.
- The speculum exam should assess for mucopurulent cervical discharge and evidence of cervicitis.
- The bimanual exam should assess for cervical motion tenderness, uterine mobility, adnexal and uterine tenderness, and an adnexal mass.
- Imaging includes pelvic ultrasound and abdomino-pelvic CT with contrast.
- Serum white blood cell count will be elevated and demonstrate a left shift, consistent with an infectious process.
- Laparoscopy may confirm a suspicious diagnosis.

Management[2]
- Laparoscopy is indicated in patients with antimicrobial failure or suspected rupture.
- Women with a tubo-ovarian abscess should be hospitalized for at least 24 hours for parenteral antibiotics and observation.
- The CDC recommends several different parenteral strategies in treating a tubo-ovarian abscess:
  - Cefotetan 2 g intravenously every 12 hours OR cefoxitin 2 g intravenously every 6 hours, PLUS doxycycline 100 mg either orally or intravenously every 8 hours

- ○ An alternative regimen is ampicillin/sulbactam 3 g intravenously every 6 hours and doxycycline 100 mg intravenously or orally every 12 hours
- ○ If the patient improves after 24 hours, clindamycin or metronidazole with doxycycline should be continued for 14 days
- ○ Parenteral antibiotics should be continued until the white blood cell count normalizes, the patient's temperature normalizes, the abscess either decreases or stays the same size, and the patient has decreased pain

REFERENCES

1. Kairys N, Roepke C. Tubo-ovarianabscess. 2018 https://www.cdc.gov/std/pid/ Updated May 4, 2019.
2. Centers for Disease Control and Prevention. Pelvic inflammatory disease. https://www.cdc.gov/std/pid/

URINARY INCONTINENCE

Etiology[1]

- The etiology of urinary incontinence in women depends largely on the type of urinary incontinence.
- In many women, hypermobility of the urethra due to pelvic support issues causes stress incontinence.
  - ○ Decreased pelvic support can occur after pregnancy, in obese women, in menopause due to lack of estrogen, and because of other genetic conditions that effect the strength of connective tissue, such as Ehlers-Danlos syndrome.

Epidemiology

- Estimates regarding incidence show that about 25% of young women, up to 57% of perimenopausal and postmenopausal women, and 75% of older women have experienced some degree of urinary incontinence.

Clinical Presentation

- The most common types of urinary incontinence in women are stress, urge, and mixed urinary incontinence (Table 2.8).
  - ○ Stress incontinence occurs when women laugh, cough, sneeze, jump, or engage in any other activity that increases intraabdominal pressure.
  - ○ Urge incontinence is the involuntary loss of urine that occurs when women feel the need to urinate. There is usually some urgency associated with the need to urinate, hence the name *urge incontinence*.
  - ○ Mixed incontinence is a combination of stress and urge incontinence.
- It is important to rule out other less common causes of urinary incontinence, including fistulas, infection, functional, and pharmacologic causes.

TABLE 2.8 Summary of the Three Most Common Types of Urinary Incontinence in Women

Type of Incontinence	Symptoms	Treatment Options
Stress incontinence	Involuntary loss of urine when laughing, coughing, sneezing, jumping, or engaging in any other activity that increases intraabdominal pressure.	Bladder training in mild disease; weight loss if obese; pelvic floor physiotherapy; pessary
Urge incontinence	Involuntary loss of urine that occurs when women feel the need to urinate. Usually accompanied by some urgency associated with the need to urinate.	Bladder training in mild disease; pelvic floor physiotherapy; antimuscarinics/anticholinergics; beta-3 agonists; onabotulinumotix A
Mixed incontinence	Presents with as a combination of the symptoms previously described.	As previously described; patients with the GUSM may benefit from vaginal estrogen

GUSM, genitourinary syndrome of menopause.

- ○ Functional urinary incontinence may occur in patients with psychiatric disorders.
- ○ Neurologic causes of urinary incontinence include cauda equina syndrome, spinal cord injury, multiple sclerosis, and Parkinson's disease.
- Overactive bladder is a condition manifested by urinary urgency with or without urinary incontinence. Many women with overactive bladder will experience nocturia and frequency of urination.
  - ○ It is important to rule out infection in patients who present with frequency of urination.
  - ○ Review the patient's medication list to rule out pharmacologic causes of frequency and nocturia including the use of diuretics.

Diagnosis

- Every patient who presents with urinary incontinence should have a thorough history taken and physical examination.
  - ○ History should address gravida and para status, reproductive age (pre- or postmenopausal), timing and duration of symptoms, pelvic instrumentation/surgery, medical conditions, prior treatment modalities, and medication review.
  - ○ Physical examination should address presence of anatomical defects and urethral mobility.
  - ○ The bimanual exam should focus on measuring pelvic floor strength and noting evidence of pelvic organ prolapse.
  - ○ A rectal examination should be performed on women to evaluate for sphincter tone, rectovaginal fistulas, masses, internal hemorrhoids, and fissures.

- ○ A neurological exam should include mental status and sensory and motor assessments of the lower extremities and perineum.
- Have the patient cough while examining the external genitalia. Loss of urine with cough is considered diagnostic for stress urinary incontinence.

> **CLINICAL PEARL:** Have extraabsorbent pads under the patient and be prepared to have protective eyewear and nonabsorbent garments to protect from urine that may spray.

- ○ Urodynamic testing may help to differentiate and quantify urinary incontinence.
- ○ Cystometry allows the quantification of bladder pressure as it relates to bladder filling and voiding, bladder sensation and capacity, and detrusor activity.
- ○ Pressure-flow and uroflowmetry studies can aid in the diagnosis of bladder voiding dysfunction.

Management

- Management depends on the type, etiology, and severity of urinary incontinence.
- Bladder training can be beneficial in patients with mild incontinence.
- Weight loss can help symptoms in women who are obese.
- Women who experience nocturia should be counseled to decrease evening fluids for a few hours before going to sleep.
- Reduction in caffeine intake may help to alleviate symptoms in mild incontinence.
- Pelvic floor physiotherapy is indicated for patients with stress, urge, and mixed urinary incontinence. It is considered a first-line treatment option.
- Certain pessaries may be helpful in women with stress urinary incontinence.
- Pharmacologic interventions are generally reserved for patients with urge incontinence. These may be useful in patients with mixed incontinence.
  - ○ Antimuscarinics/anticholinergics are the oldest drugs used for incontinence. There are oral and transdermal preparations available. Common side effects include dry mouth and dry eyes.
  - ○ Beta-3 agonists are one of the newer classes of drugs for urinary incontinence.
  - ○ Onabotulinumotix A can be injected into the bladder mucosa.
  - ○ Vaginal estradiol should be used in patients with the genitourinary syndrome of menopause if no contraindications to estrogen exist.
- Invasive interventions include urethral bulking agents, midurethral mesh slings, Burch colposuspension, and autologous bladder neck slings.
  - ○ Urethral bulking agents are injected periurethrally in women who have stress incontinence.

○ The most common surgical intervention for stress incontinence is the placement of a synthetic midurethral mesh sling.
○ If patients have concomitant pelvic organ prolapse, other interventions may be appropriate as well.

REFERENCE

1. American College of Obstetricians and Gynecologists. ACOG Practice Bulletin no. 155. Urinary incontinence in women. https://www.acog.org/Clinical-Guidance-and-Publications/Practice-Bulletins/Committee-on-Practice-Bulletins-Gynecology/Urinary-Incontinence-in-Women. Published November 2015. Reaffirmed 2018.

URINARY TRACT INFECTION

Etiology[1]

- UTIs, including cystitis, are almost always caused by bacteria.
- *Escherichia coli* is the most commonly identified bacteria in urine cultures.
- Some women will develop a UTI due to chlamydia or yeast.
- Sexual activity is a risk factor for the development of UTIs.
- Women with the GUSM may develop UTIs.
- Uncomplicated UTIs are infections that occur in otherwise healthy patients.
- Complicated UTIs include multi-drug-resistant infections, abnormalities of the genitourinary tract, and immunocompromise.

Epidemiology

- About six million women seek medical attention every year for a UTI.
- Asymptomatic bacteriuria is present in up to 10% of pregnant women.

Clinical Presentation

- Common symptoms include burning with urination, frequency of urination, gross hematuria, flank pain, suprapubic tenderness, and bladder fullness.
- Patients may have fever and chills but these symptoms are more likely to be present in patients with pyelonephritis.
- Patients may have a concomitant vaginal discharge. These patients must have a pelvic exam.

Diagnosis

- A careful history and physical exam are essential when evaluating a patient with symptoms suggestive of a UTI.
- Patients with prolonged symptoms who are not toxic appearing may have interstitial cystitis.

- The physical examination should include a mental status examination, temperature, blood pressure, respiratory rate, and pulse rate.
  - ○ Older patients with UTIs can present with an acute onset of altered mental status. Immunocompromised and hospitalized patients can develop urosepsis.
- The physical examination should also include a pelvic exam to evaluate the presence of vaginal discharge or vulvar lesions.
  - ○ Patients with a primary vulvar herpes outbreak may present with the chief complaint of dysuria.
- Urine dipstick may show hematuria, leukocyte esterase, and nitrites.
- Hematuria without signs and symptoms suggestive of a UTI may occur in patients who are actively menstruating.
- Leukocyte esterase is 57% to 96% sensitive and 94% to 98% specific for pyuria.
- Nitrites can be positive in patients with *Proteus* and *E. coli* infections.
  - ○ Urinary nitrites are 22% sensitive and 94% to 100% specific for pyuria.
- Urine culture that shows 1,000 CFU/mL in a clean-catch urine sample is diagnostic of UTI.
  - ○ A urine culture is not always necessary if the patient has signs and symptoms of an uncomplicated UTI.
- Colonization with >10,000 CFU/mL of a known uropathogen in an otherwise asymptomatic patient is diagnostic for asymptomatic bacteriuria.

Management

- See Table 2.9 for an overview of the treatment of UTIs in pregnant and nonpregnant patients.
- Asymptomatic bacteriuria in a pregnant patient is associated with preterm labor, intrauterine growth restriction, amnionitis, and low-birth-weight babies. As such, it must be treated.
  - ○ Antimicrobial options in pregnancy include nitrofurantoin, fosfomycin, ampicillin, cephalexin, and amoxicillin–clavulanic acid.
  - ○ Trimethoprim/sulfamethoxazole should be avoided during the first or third trimesters.

TABLE 2.9 Treatment Options for Uncomplicated UTI

Nonpregnant*	Pregnant
Nitrofurantoin	Nitrofurantoin
Fosfomycin	Fosfomycin
Ampicillin	Ampicillin
Cephalexin	Cephalexin
Amoxicillin–clavulanic acid	Amoxicillin–clavulanic acid
Trimethoprim/sulfamethoxazole	

*Avoid the use of fluoroquinolones, particularly as a first-line choice.
UTI, urinary tract infection.

- ○ Remember that most organisms are Gram negative so appropriate antimicrobials should reflect the most common etiologies and known sensitivity and resistance patterns.
- Uncomplicated UTIs in nonpregnant patients can be treated with the same antimicrobials as in pregnancy, with the addition of trimethoprim/sulfamethoxazole.
- Duration of treatment varies, from 1 day with fosfomycin to 7 to 10 days with other antimicrobials.
  - ○ There is evidence that 3 to 5 days of treatment are sufficient in uncomplicated UTIs.
- The urinary analgesic phenazopyridine can be used in nonpregnant patients with uncomplicated UTIs.
  - ○ Advise patients that their urine will turn an orange-red color while using phenazopyridine.
  - ○ Patients should not use phenazopyridine for longer than a few days.

CLINICAL PEARL: Hematuria in asymptomatic patients who are not menstruating could indicate malignancy.

REFERENCE

1. Brusch JL. Urinary tract infection (UTI) and cystitis (bladder infection) in females. In: Bronze MS, ed. *Medscape*. https://emedicine.medscape.com/article/233101-overview. Updated July 19, 2019.

VAGINITIS

Etiology

- The most common organisms associated with infectious vaginitis are *Candida* species (*Candida albicans* and *Candida glabrata*), bacterial vaginosis (BV; *Garderella vaginalis* is the most common bacteria), and trichomoniasis (*Trichomonas vaginalis*).

Epidemiology

- BV is the most common cause of infectious vaginitis in women who present to their healthcare providers.[1]
- It is difficult to assess the incidence of vaginal candidiasis due to the widespread availability of over-the-counter antifungal medications,
- Although trichomoniasis is a sexually transmitted disease, it is not reportable, so prevalence is difficult to estimate.

Clinical Presentation

- Patients complain of vaginal discharge that may have associated pruritus, vaginal burning, dyspareunia, and malodor.
- On physical exam, vaginal discharge is present.
- Candidal discharge is usually thick, white, and clumpy. The vulva can be affected as well, with small fissures and erythema present.
- BV typically presents as a thin, off-white or grayish vaginal discharge with an amine odor (fishy smell) that can worsen with sexual intercourse, and is present when mixed with 10% potassium hydroxide (KOH).
- Trichomoniasis is usually a greenish-yellow, frothy, thin discharge. The cervix can be affected, showing punctations and erythema, commonly referred to as *strawberry cervix.*
- The vaginal pH is elevated in BV and trichomoniasis (>4.5).

Diagnosis

- There are several diagnostic modalities.
- Wet prep is the least expensive testing option but is less sensitive and specific than other available options.
- Budding yeast, hyphae, and pseudohyphae under KOH microscopy indicate candida.
- Clue cells indicate BV, and motile flagellated organisms indicate trichomoniasis.
- The Amsel Criteria for BV include a thin white or yellow discharge, a pH greater than 4.5, and clue cells on saline microscopy.
- There are several commercial testing modalities for infectious vaginitis that can be used if available.
- See Figure 2.4.

Management[1]

- See Table 2.10 for an overview of the treatment of vaginitis.
- Treatment of symptomatic candida infections include azole antifungal vaginal creams and suppositories, and oral fluconazole.
- Most women prefer the oral fluconazole to creams and suppositories, but it is important to let women know that oral azoles can take up to 2 days longer than topicals to achieve symptom improvement.
- Resistant cases of vaginal candidiasis can occur and are usually due to *Candida glabrata.*
  ○ Oral fluconazole 150 mg by mouth with three sequential doses 72 hours apart is usually sufficient treatment.
- The preferred treatment of BV is with either vaginal or oral metronidazole.
- Vaginal metronidazole is dosed daily for 5 days.
- Oral metronidazole dosing is 500 mg twice daily for 7 days.
- Metronidazole can cause an antabuse effect if the patient ingests alcohol, so specific patient education on alcohol abstinence during treatment must occur.

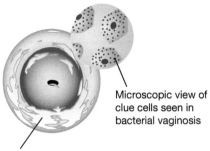

Microscopic view of
clue cells seen in
bacterial vaginosis

(a) View of cervix through speculum

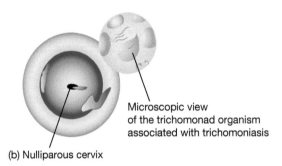

Microscopic view
of the trichomonad organism
associated with trichomoniasis

(b) Nulliparous cervix

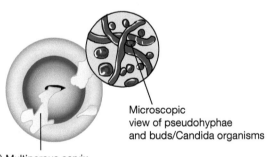

Microscopic
view of pseudohyphae
and buds/Candida organisms

(c) Multiparous cervix

Figure 2.4 (a) View of the cervix through a speculum. (b) Nulliparous
cervix. (c) Multiparous cervix.
Source: Secor RM, Fantasia HC. *Fast Facts About the Gynecologic Exam.* 2nd ed. New
York, NY: Springer Publishing Company; 2018:50.

- An alternative to metronidazole for BV is oral or vaginal clindamycin.
  - As BV is associated with premature rupture of membranes, low birth
    weight, and prematurity, it is important to treat pregnant patients.

TABLE 2.10 Overview of the Treatment of Vaginitis

Condition	Antimicrobial	Notes
Bacterial vaginosis	Metronidazole (oral or vaginal)	Metronidazole can cause an antabuse effect; do not use alcohol.
	Clindamycin (oral or vaginal)	Although clindamycin has been implicated in *Clostridium difficile* diarrheal infection, almost all antimicrobials can cause CDI.
Trichomoniasis	Metroniazole (oral) or tinidazole (oral)	Metronidazole and tinidazole can cause an antabuse effect; do not use alcohol.
		Sexual contacts must be treated.
Candidiasis	Fluconazole (oral) or topical azole antifungal cream or suppository	Resistant candidal infections can be treated with oral fluconazole 150 mg by mouth with three sequential doses 72 hours apart.
		Use with caution in patients with renal or hepatic disease, or those who are proarrythmic as QT prolongation has occurred.

CDI, *Clostridium difficile* infection.

- Trichomoniasis is treated with oral metronidazole or tinidazole, 2 g by mouth in one dose.
- Sexual partners must be treated as well.
  - As with BV, trichomoniasis is also associated with premature rupture of membranes, low birth weight, and prematurity, so it is important to treat pregnant patients.
  - Oral metronidazole is advised.
  - Tinidazole is not advised in pregnancy.

> **CLINICAL PEARL:** Patients with recurrent yeast infections should be screened for diabetes and immunodeficiency.

REFERENCE

1. American College of Obstetricians and Gynecologists. ACOG practice bulletin no. 72. Vaginitis. https://www.acog.org/Clinical-Guidance-and-Publications/Practice-Bulletins/Committee-on-Practice-Bulletins-Gynecology/Vaginitis. Published May 2006. Reaffirmed 2019.

VULVAR CONDYLOMA

Etiology

- About 90% of vulvar condylomas are nononcogenic HPV 6 and 11.[1]
- Particularly in patients with HIV, oncogenic HPV strains can be identified, including 16, 18, 31, 33, and 35.[2]

- Oncogenic strains 16 and 18 are the most common in the United States.[2]
- Oncogenic strains are associated with high-grade vulvar epithelial lesions.[2]

Epidemiology[1]

- Prevalence is estimated at over 50%.
- Patients who are immunocompromised tend to have more severe disease.
- Patients who have previously been asymptomatic may develop active disease during pregnancy.
- Risk factors include tobacco smoking, multiple sexual partners, and early age at first intercourse.

Clinical Presentation[1,2]

- Symptomatic patients may have pruritus or discomfort.
- Classic lesions are described as cauliflower-like but may also appear as papular, fleshy raised lesions (verrucous), lobulated, or plaques.
- Number and size of lesions can vary from a small, single lesion to complete obliteration of the introitus.

Diagnosis

- Diagnosis is accomplished with physical examination and inspection of the vulva, perineum, and anus.
- Suspicious lesions, lesions that seem to worsen with treatment, and bleeding or ulcerated lesions should be biopsied to rule out malignancy.[2]

Management[2]

- Topical options include imiquimod, podophyllum, podofilox, trichloroacetic acid, sinecatechins, and cryotherapy.
- Patient-applied options
  - Imiquimod 5% cream is applied nightly, three nights a week, for up to 16 weeks
    - Imiquimod should not be used in pregnant women due to lack of safety data.
  - Podofilox 0.5% gel or solution is applied twice daily for 3 days, off for 4 days, with a repeat of the cycle for four cycles
    - Podofilox use is not recommend in pregnant women.
  - A weekly application of podophyllum resin 10% to 25% should be appliedcarefully to avoid unaffected areas
    - Podophyllum resin should be washed off the treated area 1 to 4 hours after application.
    - Podophyllum resin should only be used for smaller lesions ; its safety in pregnancy has not been established.
  - Sinecatechins 15% ointment can be applied three times a day for up to 16 weeks.
    - Sinecatechin safety during pregnancy has not been established.

- Provider-applied options
  - ○ Trichloroacetic acid can be applied sparingly to lesions with care not to apply to unaffected tissue
    - ■ Trichloroacetic acid can be used weekly and its safety in pregnancy has not been established.
  - ○ Cryotherapy
- Surgical regimens include cauterization and laser ablation.
- Cesarean delivery may be considered in women with extensive disease that obstructs the pelvic outlet and in women with friable lesions that could cause excessive bleeding with vaginal delivery.
- Prevention of HPV is accomplished with the recombinant 9-valent HPV vaccine.

REFERENCES

1. Ghadishah, D. Condyloma acuminatum(genital warts). In: Brenner BE, ed. *Medscape*. https://emedicine.medscape.com/article/781735-overview. Updated October 22, 2018.
2. Workowski KA, Bolan GA. Sexually transmitted diseases treatment guidelines, 2015. *MMWR Recomm Rep*. 2015;64(3). https://www.cdc.gov/std/tg2015/tg-2015-print.pdf

VULVAR INTRAEPITHELIAL NEOPLASIA AND VULVAR CARCINOMA

Etiology[1]

- Vulvar intraephilial neoplasia (VIN) and vulvar carcinoma are two distinct entities.
- VIN is divided into low grade, high grade, and differentiated lesions. Low-grade and high-grade lesions are due to HPV.
- Differentiated VIN usually occurs in postmenopausal women with a history of lichen sclerosis. It is associated with progression to vulvar squamous cell carcinoma.
- Vulvar carcinomas are usually squamous cell, but a small proportion can be melanoma, basal cell, Paget's disease of the vulva, or sarcoma.

Epidemiology

- VIN is increasing in incidence, with the largest burden of disease reported among women in their 40s.[1]
- Tobacco use is strongly correlated with high-grade VIN. Women should be advised on tobacco cessation.[1]
- Vulvar cancer accounts for approximately 0.6% of reproductive cancers in women.[2]

Clinical Presentation

- Low-grade and high-grade lesions can be asymptomatic, found incidentally on examination of the vulva.
- High-grade lesions are more likely to present with vulvar pruritus and pain/burning.
- Vulvar lesions can appear white, gray, red, or brown, and are often raised. They can be plaques, nodules, or papules.
- It can be difficult to differentiate between a benign verrucous lesion and VIN, squamous cell carcinoma, and lichen sclerosis/lichen planus, thus any suspicious lesion should be biopsied.
- Vulvar carcinoma presents with a vulvar lesion accompanied by pruritus and/or bleeding.

Diagnosis[1]

- Diagnosis is made histologically with vulvar biopsy.
- Any lesion that has been treated as a benign verruca but does not resolve must be biopsied.
- Women who present with unremitting pruritus despite treatment for candidiasis, condyloma, or lichen sclerosis, should have a vulvar colposcopy.
- Any irregularities found on colposcopy should be biopsied, and on occasion, even areas without visible abnormalities may be considered for biopsy when the patient remains symptomatic.

Management[1]

- Management of low-grade lesions should be treated the same as a condyloma.
- Low-grade lesions are not precancerous, so patient reassurance is essential.
- The treatment of high-grade lesions depends on the histology, extent of disease, and other risk factors, such as tobacco use, age older than 45 years, immunosuppression, and history of lichen sclerosis.
- Wide excision is preferred for all patients with high-grade lesions.
- Other options include vulvectomy, laser ablation, and topical therapy.
- Topical therapies include imiquimod and fluoroucil. Cidofovir is being investigated as a possible topical treatment.
- Differentiated VIN has a strong association with invasive vulvar carcinoma and should be excised.
- Retrospective data suggest that a significant portion of women with high-grade or differentiated VIN will be found to have invasive vulvar carcinoma on excision specimens.
- The treatment of vulvar cancer is radical vulvectomy; inguinofemoral lymphadenectomy is determined by lymphovascular involvement and size of the tumor.
- Radiation therapy is recommended if more than one lymph node is positive.
- Metastatic disease is treated with cisplatin or a cisplatin combination.[3]

> **CLINICAL PEARL:** Any woman with persistent vulvar pruritus should undergo vulvar colposcopy with biopsy.

REFERENCES

1. American College of Obstetricians and Gynecologists. ACOG committee opinion no. 675. Management of vulvar intraepithelial neoplasia. https://www.acog.org/Clinical-Guidance-and-Publications/Committee-Opinions/Committee-on Gynecologic-Practice/Management-of-Vulvar-Intraepithelial-Neoplasia. Published October 2016. Reaffirmed 2019.
2. American Cancer Society. Key statistics for vulvar cancer. https://www.cancer.org/cancer/vulvar-cancer/about/key-statistics.html. Updated January 9, 2019.
3. Jewell EL. Vulvar cancer treatment protocols. In: Sonoda Y, ed. *Medscape.* https://emedicine.medscape.com/article/2156990-overview. Updated January 20, 2017.

VULVODYNIA

Etiology[1,2]

- The etiology of vulvodynia is poorly understood but may be related to several issues, including hypersensitivity of nerves, inflammation by cytokines, and pelvic floor dysfunction.
- The most common location of pain is the vulvar vestibule.
- The vulvar vestibule is an area of tissue that separates the internal reproductive tract from the external labia minora and majora (Figure 2.5).

Epidemiology[1,2]

- Estimates of incidence vary from 7% to 16%.

Clinical Presentation[1,2]

- Patients will present with vulvar pain of at least 3 months' duration without an identifiable cause.

Diagnosis

- Vulvodynia is a diagnosis of exclusion.
- History should address comorbidities, including endometriosis, interstitial cystitis, and any chronic pain syndrome.
- History should also address the patient's emotional status, sexual function, and any other related psychosocial issues.

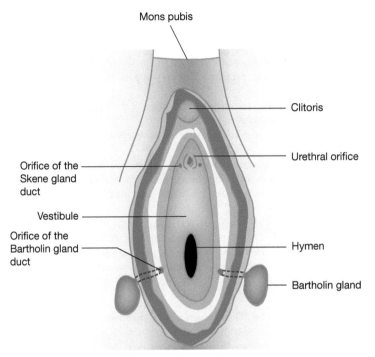

FIGURE 2.5   Anatomy of the vestibular glands.

- Other pathologies that need to be ruled out include the following:
  - Infectious etiologies, such as candidiasis and herpes simplex virus
  - Malignancy, such as squamous cell cancer or melanoma
  - Trauma, such as female genital cutting/mutilation
  - Inflammation, such as lichen planus, lichen sclerosis, lichen simplex, and contact dermatitis
  - Neurological etiologies, such as nerve trauma and neuropathy
  - GSUM
  - Iatrogenic, such as radiation therapy
- Inspection of the vulva, vulvar vestibule, and perineum should be performed.
- A cotton swab test involves asking the patient to point to where the pain is located, and then ,.beginning at the inner thigh, touch the patient with the cotton swab, gradually moving medially and making sure to assess the vulva, clitoris, perineum, and the vestibule itself.[3]
  - The patient should report her level of pain or discomfort at each area.
- A pinprick test should follow the same procedure as the cotton swab test.[3]
- Localized provoked vulvodynia (LPV, or provoked vulvodynia [PV]) is a disorder that causes chronic pain at the vulvar vestibule.[2,3]

- LPV can be differentiated from general vulvodynia in that LPV is a burning, sharp pain that persists after light pressure has been applied to the area.[3]
- Assess the pelvic floor musculature by having the patient perform a Kegel maneuver while the examiner's finger is just past the hymenal ring in the vagina.
- Bimanual examination consists of palpation of the ischial spines; bladder and urethra; and uterus and adnexa.
  - Women with pudendal neuralgia will exhibit pain with palpation of the ischial spines.[2]
  - Women with interstitial cystitis may exhibit pain with palpation of the urethra, the area just below the urethra, or the bladder neck.[2]
  - Palpation of the uterus and adnexa are done to rule out any other pelvic pathology.
- Women with general vulvodynia will often present with daily pain that is unprovoked.[2]
- Women with provoked vulvodynia will present with pain upon entry of the vagina and pain with vestibular palpation or pressure.[2]

Management

- Management can be difficult when there is no underlying known pathology.
- It is essential to validate the patient's pain even in the absence of visual abnormalities.
- Address the patient's concerns regarding quality-of-life issues, particularly sexuality.
- Principles of management include the following:
  - Avoid vulvar irritants, such as soaps.
  - Tricyclic antidepressants, serotonin-norepinephrine reuptake inhibitors, and some antiseizure medications, such as gabapentin and topiramate, have been used with various levels of success and as such, the evidence is weak to support its routine use.[2]
  - Compounded topical agents include combinations of lidocaine, gabapentin, estrogen, and testosterone.[1]
  - There is no strong evidence that hormonal creams or steroid creams are effective in premenopausal women.[2]
  - Localized estrogen, particularly estrogen applied directly to the vulva/vestibule, may alleviate symptoms in peri- and postmenopausal women.[2]
  - Women should maintain adequate moisture of the vulva by using an approved hypoallergenic vulvar ointment or cream.[2]
  - A physiotherapist who specializes in pelvic floor dysfunction and chronic pelvic pain can be of assistance.
  - Referral to sexual counselors may be appropriate in women who report loss of sexual function.

○ Sometimes women benefit from the use of vaginal dilators.
○ A multidisciplinary approach to holistic treatment should be utilized.

REFERENCES

1. Faye RB, Piraccini E. Vulvodynia [Internet]. In: *StatPearls*. Treasure Island, FL: StatPearls Publishing; 2019. https://www.ncbi.nlm.nih.gov/books/NBK430792
2. Sadownik LA. Etiology, diagnosis, and management of vulvodynia. *Int J Womens Health*. 2014;6:437–449. doi:10.2147/IJWH.S37660
3. Farmer MA. What is special about the vulvar vestibule? *Pain*. 2015;156(3):359–360. doi:10.1097/j.pain.0000000000000094

3

Common Disease Entities in Obstetrics

ABRUPTIO PLACENTAE (PLACENTAL ABRUPTION)

Etiology

- An abrupted placenta occurs when there is rupture of the decidua basalis maternal vessels along the placental villi, causing an accumulation of blood between the decidua and its attachment to the uterus.
- Some of the major risk factors include prior history of abruption, maternal trauma to the abdomen, hypertensive disorders, cocaine use, methamphetamine use, and a short umbilical cord.
- Other risk factors include tobacco use, premature rupture of membranes, and acute decompression in a patient with polyhydramnios.

Epidemiology

- Placental abruption occurs in about one in 120 births and is a leading cause of maternal and fetal death.[1]
- Disseminated intravascular coagulopathy (DIC) is present in about 20% of severe abruptions, and abruption is the leading cause of DIC in pregnancy.[1]

Clinical Presentation

- Patients typically present with acute abdominal pain, vaginal bleeding, and uterine contractions.
- Vaginal bleeding is present in 80% of abruptio placentae patients.[1]

- Vaginal bleeding may not be present if the hemorrhage is concealed in the fundus.
- Hypotension and fetal heart rate abnormalities are more strongly correlated than amount of bleeding with degree of abruption and potential maternal and fetal death.

Diagnosis

- The diagnosis is made clinically. Any patient who presents with painful vaginal bleeding and uterine tenderness should be considered abrupted until proven otherwise.
- Ultrasonography may reveal a placenta previa but the diagnosis should never be ruled out based on a normal ultrasound.
- A retroplacental hematoma is the classic finding of abruptio placentae but may be present in only 2% of patients with abruptions.[1]

Management

- Small abruptions can be managed medically with antenatal steroids, if gestation age is less than 34 weeks and the patient and fetus are clinically stable.
- Patients should be hospitalized for at least 48 hours with continuous fetal heart rate monitoring and ongoing evaluation of maternal status.
- The management of a significant abruption requires a multidisciplinary team approach in the labor and delivery suite of the hospital. See Chapter 6, Urgent Management of OB/GYN Conditions.
- Further management depends on the age of gestation and presence or absence of hypovolemia or other severe features, such as DIC.
- For stable patients at gestational age less than 32 weeks, magnesium sulfate may be given for neuroprotection; for gestational age less than 34 weeks antenatal steroids should be considered.
- Group B *Streptococcus* prophylaxis should also be considered.
- Cesarean delivery is almost always indicated unless vaginal delivery is imminent.

> **CLINICAL PEARL:** Vaginal bleeding may be sparse or hemorrhagic, but the amount of bleeding does not correlate well with the size of placental abruption.

REFERENCE

1. Hobel CJ, Lamb AR. Obstetric hemorrhage. In: Hacker NF, Gambone JC, Hobel CJ, eds. *Hacker and Moore's Essentials of Obstetrics and Gynecology.* 6th ed. Philadelphia, PA: Saunders/Elsevier; 2016:136–146.

ANEMIA

Etiology

- The physiologic changes associated with pregnancy include increased iron demands, increased total red blood cell mass, and a total blood volume expansion causing a mild dilutional anemia, which is a physiologic process.
- Most anemia in pregnancy in the absence of underlying disorders is an acquired iron-deficiency anemia.
- Iron-deficiency anemia in pregnancy is associated with preterm delivery, increased perinatal mortality, and low birth weight.
- There may be an association between iron-deficiency anemia in pregnancy and adverse developmental outcomes in children.

Epidemiology

- Pregnant teenage patients have the highest prevalence of anemia in the United States.
- When anemia is classified as a hemoglobin level less than 10 g/dL, prevalence is 21.55 per 1,000 women.

Clinical Presentation

- Most women will be asymptomatic.
- Signs and symptoms of anemia are the same as in nonpregnant women but overlap with many of the common symptoms in pregnancy, such as being easily fatigued and mild shortness of breath.
- Some women will develop pica syndrome (eating nonfood items, such as soil and paper) during pregnancy. Pica is associated with iron-deficiency anemia.

Diagnosis

- The diagnosis of anemia in pregnancy requires a thorough history and physical exam to rule out underlying pathology.
- Laboratory testing for anemia includes hemoglobin, hematocrit, red blood cell indices such as mean corpuscular volume (MCV), serum iron, total iron binding capacity, and serum ferritin levels.
- In patients with a suspected hemoglobinopathy, it may be appropriate to order a hemoglobin electrophoresis.
- In patients with low hemoglobin and hematocrit, always evaluate the MCV so that you can classify the patient as being microcytic, macrocytic, or normocytic.
- Low MCV (microcytic) is associated with the following:
  - Iron-deficiency anemia
  - Thalassemias

- High MCV (macrocytic) is associated with the following:
  - Folic acid deficiency
  - B12 deficiency
  - Hemolytic anemia due to prescribed drugs, such as certain antiretrovirals for HIV
  - Chronic alcohol abuse
  - Hepatic disease
- Normal MCV (normocytic) is associated with the following:
  - Early iron-deficiency anemia
  - Anemia of chronic disease
  - Anemia in hypothyroidism
  - Hemorrhagic conditions
  - Bone marrow suppression
  - Chronic renal disease
- American College of Obstetricians and Gynecologists (ACOG) uses the following hemoglobin and hematocrit values to diagnose anemia in pregnancy:[1]
  - Hemoglobin
    - <11 g/dL in the first trimester
    - <10.5 g/dL in the second trimester
    - <11 g/dL in the third trimester
  - Hematocrit
    - <33% in the first trimester
    - <32% in the second trimester
    - <33% in the third trimester
- Decreased serum iron indicates iron-deficiency anemia
- Increased total iron binding capacity indicates iron deficiency anemia
- Decreased ferritin indicates iron deficiency anemia
- A serum ferritin ≤30 ng/mL is diagnostic of iron deficiency anemia
- Hemoglobin and hematocrit levels tend to be lower among women of color

Management
- Iron-deficiency anemia is managed with iron supplementation.
- There are various oral iron supplements available.
  - Ferrous sulfate is a common supplement. Each 325 mg tablet contains 65 mg of elemental iron.
  - Ferrous fumarate contains 106 mg of elemental iron in each 325 mg tablet.
  - Ferrous gluconate contains 34 mg of elemental iron in each 300 mg tablet.
  - Ferrous gluconate tends to be easier on the stomach when women experience gastrointestinal (GI) upset with other iron products.
- Patients who cannot tolerate oral iron products or who are not responding may be considered for parenteral iron.

- Oral iron products can cause or exacerbate constipation, so patients should be counseled.
- Remind patients to avoid any dairy products or calcium supplements within 1 hour before or 2 hours after taking their iron supplements.
- Patients with hemoglobin less than 6 g/dL should be referred for blood transfusion as hemoglobin levels that low are associated with oligohydramnios, fetal cerebral abnormalities, and fetal demise.

> **CLINICAL PEARL:** Remind patients to take their iron supplements with vitamin C as it will enhance absorption.

REFERENCE

1. American College of Obstetricians and Gynecologists. ACOG practice bulletin no. 95. Anemia in pregnancy. https://www.acog.org/Clinical-Guidance -and-Publications/Practice-Bulletins/Committee-on-Practice-Bulletins-Obstetrics/ Anemia-in-Pregnancy. Published July 2008. Reaffirmed 2017.

ASTHMA IN PREGNANCY

Etiology
- Asthma is manifested by coughing, wheezing, and dyspnea as a result of bronchial inflammation and hyperresponsiveness to certain triggers.

Epidemiology
- Asthma complicates up to 8% of pregnancies.[1]

Clinical Presentation
- Patients may present for their initial prenatal visit and be asymptomatic, but careful history reveals asthma.
- Patients who present with an acute exacerbation should be managed according to standard practice with the use of beta agonists and corticosteroids as necessary.

Diagnosis
- Diagnosis can be based on a prior history of asthma.
- Diagnosis of asthma in pregnancy is the same as in the nonpregnant patient.
- Spirometry that reveals reversible airway obstruction as defined by greater than 12% increase in forced expiratory volume (FEV1) after inhaled bronchodilation.
- Patients may have wheezing on auscultation of the lungs, particularly when they are having an exacerbation.

Management

- Management is aimed at ensuring adequate oxygenation of the mother and fetus.
- Prematurity, preeclampsia, intrauterine growth restriction (IUGR), and cesarean delivery are risks of poorly controlled asthma.
- Long- and short-acting beta agonists are the mainstay of asthma therapy and are generally considered safe during pregnancy.
- Short-acting beta agonists, such as albuterol, should be used as rescue therapy.
- Inhaled corticosteroids should be used in patients who are not well controlled with rescue inhalers.
- In patients with mild persistent asthma, use of low-dose inhaled corticosteroids is recommended.
- In patients with mild or moderate persistent asthma, leukotriene inhibitors can be used.
- If asthma symptoms are not controlled with low-dose inhaled corticosteroids, medium-dose inhaled corticosteroids plus albuterol is recommended.
- Patients who use inhaled corticosteroids should be reminded to rinse their mouths out after each use to avoid oral candidiasis.
- Severe asthma should be treated with all of the options mentioned previously; systemic corticosteroids should also be considered.
- In patients with severe asthma, consider serial ultrasounds beginning at 32 weeks to assess fetal growth and activity.[1]
- All daily asthma medications should be continued for the duration of pregnancy and the postpartum period.
- Influenza vaccination is recommended in pregnancy and is particularly important in pregnant patients with asthma.
  - Influenza nasal spray vaccines are not recommended in pregnancy.
- In patients with asthma who are sensitive or allergic to aspirin, avoid using indomethacin as it can also induce bronchospasm.
- Magnesium sulfate, used in patients with preeclampsia with severe features and eclampsia, is a bronchodilator.

> **Clinical Pearl:** Patients with asthma should not be given nonselective beta blockers, ergonovine, or carboprost due to their bronchospastic potential.

Reference

1. American College of Obstetricians and Gynecologists. ACOG practice bulletin no. 90. Asthma in pregnancy. https://www.acog.org/Clinical-Guidance-and -Publications/Practice-Bulletins/Committee-on-Practice-Bulletins-Obstetrics/ Asthma-in-Pregnancy. Published February 2008. Reaffirmed 2019.

CERVICAL INSUFFICIENCY

Etiology[1,2]
- The etiology of cervical insufficiency, previously known as *incompetent cervix*, is unknown, but a history of cervical trauma has been implicated.
- Women with a history of cervical conization and loop electrosurgical excision procedures (LEEPs) are at greater risk of developing cervical insufficiency.

Epidemiology[1]
- The estimated incidence of cervical insufficiency is 1%.

Clinical Presentation
- Cervical insufficiency is a painless dilation of the cervix during the second trimester of a singleton pregnancy.

Diagnosis[2]
- Diagnosis is made based on a history of second-trimester delivery in a singleton pregnancy, usually before 24 weeks, in the absence of preterm labor symptoms, such as uterine contractions, and in the absence of infection or known trauma.
- ACOG states that patients with a history of a preterm delivery before 34 weeks and a cervical length less than 25 mm on ultrasound prior to 23 weeks' gestation can be considered for cerclage placement.
- Patients with a history of cerclage placement due to the prior criteria are also candidates for cerclage with subsequent pregnancies.
- Patients with a short cervix on ultrasound but no history of second-trimester delivery are not categorized as having cervical insufficiency. These patients may be candidates for vaginal progesterone.

Management[1,2]
- Testing for gonorrhea and chlamydia is essential, as is abstaining from sexual intercourse.
- Elective cerclage, in which a purse-strong suture is placed in the cervix, is done between 12 and 14 weeks' gestation in women with a history suggestive of cervical insufficiency.
- Rarely are cerclages performed after 23 weeks' gestation.
- If the cervical length is less than 25 mm by 24 weeks' gestation in a high-risk woman, cerclage can be considered.
- Removal of the cerclage is recommended at 36 to 37 weeks' gestation.
- Studies are currently underway to assess the utility of vaginal pessaries to prevent preterm delivery.

> **Clinical Pearl:** Women with a history suggestive of cervical insufficiency can have serial ultrasounds during which the cervical length is measured.

References

1. Brown R, Gagnon R, Delisle M-F. Cervical insufficiency and cervical cerclage. *J Obstet Gynaecol Can.* 2013;35(12):1115–1127. doi:10.1016/S1701-2163(15)30764-7
2. American College of Obstetricians and Gynecologists. Practice bulletin no. 142. Cerclage for the management of cervical insufficiencyhttps://www.acog.org/Clinical-Guidance-and-Publications/Practice-Bulletins/Committee-on-Practice-Bulletins-Obstetrics/Cerclage-for-the-Management-of-Cervical-Insufficiency.aspx. Published February 2014. Reaffirmed 2019.

Cholestasis of Pregnancy

Etiology

- The pathophysiology of cholestasis of pregnancy is due to the inability to secrete bile salts.
- About 15% of patients with cholestasis of pregnancy have a gene mutation.[1]
- The symptoms of cholestasis of pregnancy are due to the accumulation of bile salts.
- Estrogen is known to cause cholestasis.
  - The high levels of estrogen that occur during late pregnancy partially explain why patients will manifest the disease late in pregnancy.
  - Patients with multiple gestations are also at risk.
  - Patients who have a history of estrogen sensitivity, particularly related to the liver, should be closely monitored.

Epidemiology

- Cholestasis of pregnancy is the most common pregnancy-related hepatic disorder.
- It most often occurs during the third trimester but can occur earlier in pregnancy.
- Cholestasis of pregnancy occurs in about 1% of pregnancies.[1]

Clinical Presentation

- Patients will present with significant pruritus.
- Pruritus usually starts on the palms of the hands and the soles of the feet and spreads to the face and trunk.
- There is usually no identifiable rash associated with the pruritus.

- Pruritus is usually worse at night.
- Some patients may become icteric.

Diagnosis[1]

- Laboratory evaluation of the patient with pruritus without an identifiable rash should include total serum bile acid, cholic acid, chenodeoxycholic acid, total bilirubin, alanine aminotransferase (ALT), aspartate aminotransferase (AST), gamma-glutamyl transferase (GGT), prothrombin time (PT)/partial thromboplastin time (PTT), and international normalized ratio (INR).
- A serum bile acid level greater than 10 micromol/L is diagnostic.
  - A serum bile acid level greater than 100 micromol/L is associated with significant mortality.
- Cholic acid is increased and chenodeoxycholic acid is slightly increased.
- The cholic acid/chenodeoxycholic acid ratio will be slightly increased.
- It may take several days for the lab to run bile acid testing.
- ALT and AST can be used while bile acid tests are pending.
  - Although levels of ALT are normally elevated during pregnancy, levels greater than 40 IU/L in the presence of pruritus can be sufficient to diagnose cholestasis of pregnancy.

Management[1]

- Severe cases of cholestasis of pregnancy can result in fat malabsorption and vitamin K deficiency, which can result in postpartum hemorrhage.
- Laboratory values should be monitored every 2 to 3 weeks until delivery.
- Patients with cholestasis of pregnancy should have serial nonstress tests (NSTs), biophysical profiles (BPPs), and possibly umbilical artery Doppler studies.
- Patients who are stable should deliver at 37 weeks.
  - If bile acids are consistently lower than 40 micromol/L and pruritus is controlled, delivery may be deferred until 38 to 39 weeks, but patients should continue to be closely monitored.
- Amniocentesis can be done to evaluate fetal lung maturity when patients are preterm.
- If amniocentesis is performed and meconium is found, delivery should occur regardless of fetal lung maturity results.
- If at any time during surveillance there is evidence of fetal compromise, delivery should occur.
- Pharmacologic management is with ursodeoxycholic acid (UDCA).
- Over-the-counter diphenhydramine can be used for pruritus.
- Hydroxyzine can be used for severe pruritus and the possible insomnia associated with an increase in nocturnal symptoms.

CLINICAL PEARL: Always keep cholestasis of pregnancy on your differential in a pregnant patient who presents with persistent pruritus.

REFERENCE

1. Rigby FB. Intrahepatic cholestasis of pregnancy. In Ramus RM, ed. *Medscape.* https://emedicine.medscape.com/article/1562288-overview. Updated December 12, 2018.

EARLY PREGNANCY LOSS/NONELECTIVE ABORTION

Etiology

- Nonelective termination of pregnancy, also called *spontaneous abortion, early pregnancy loss (EPL),* or *miscarriage,* is defined as a pregnancy loss prior to 20 weeks' gestation.
- Most cases of nonelective abortions occur prior to 13 weeks' gestation.
- The term *early pregnancy loss* is often used to define a nonviable intrauterine pregnancy within the first 12w6d gestation (Box 3.1).

Epidemiology[1]

- Spontaneous and threatened abortions are one of the most common first trimester pregnancy complications.
- Modifiable risk factors include cigarette smoking; illicit drug use, particularly amphetamines such as cocaine; and extremes of maternal body weight.
- Most miscarriages occur due to fetal chromosomal abnormalities.
- EPL can occur in about 10% of pregnancies, and 80% of pregnancy losses occur in the first trimester.

Box 3.1 Ultrasound Findings in Early Pregnancy Loss

Intrauterine pregnancy with a gestational sac and embryo or fetus, but no fetal cardiac activity OR An empty gestational sac by 12w6d gestation
Mean gestational sac of ≥25 mm AND No embryo AND Crown–rump length ≥7 mm with no cardiac activity

Source: American College of Obstetricans and Gynecologists. Practice bulletin no. 200. Early pregnancy loss. https://www.acog.org/Clinical-Guidance-and-Publications/Practice-Bulletins/Committee-on-Practice-Bulletins-Gynecology/Early-Pregnancy-Loss. Published August 29, 2018.

Clinical Presentation

- Patients will usually present with first-trimester bleeding with or without pelvic pain or cramping.
- Sometimes women will pass tissue, or products of conception.

Diagnosis[1]

- A careful history and physical exam must document the last menstrual period, gravida and para status, presence or absence of risk factors, and an assessment of hemodynamic status.
- Any signs of hemodynamic instability require emergent management.
- The pelvic examination should assess for vaginal bleeding, cervical dilation, cervical tenderness, size and mobility of the uterus, and any palpable masses.
- Transvaginal ultrasonography is most helpful to check for the presence of a gestational sac, fetal pole, fetal heart tones, retained products of conception, fluid in the cul-de-sac, or adnexal masses.
- Laboratory analyses include a quantitative beta human chorionic gonadotropin (beta-HCG), serum progesterone, complete blood count (CBC), Rh status, and type and cross.
    - A disseminated intravascular coagulation (DIC) panel may be warranted in specific situations, such as heavy bleeding.
- Ultrasound findings highly suggestive of EPL are an intrauterine pregnancy with a gestational sac and embryo or fetus, but no fetal cardiac activity, or an empty gestational sac by 12w6d gestation.
- The Society of Radiologists in Ultrasound have developed criteria for EPL.
    - These include mean gestational sac of greater than or equal to 25 mm and no embryo and crown–rump length greater than or equal to 7 mm with no cardiac activity.[2]
- Sometimes fetal bradycardia less than 100 bpm and a subchorionic hemorrhage are found, but in and of themselves are not diagnostic of EPL.

Management[1]

- Management is dependent upon each situation.
- Expectant management is appropriate for some women who are hemodynamically stable, show no signs of infection, and are less than 13w6d gestation.
- In women with a complete abortion, no treatment is necessary unless the patient is Rh (D) negative or still bleeding.
- Rh (D)-negative women should be given Rho (D) immune globulin within 72 hours.
- Bleeding can sometimes be managed with the addition of methylergonovine 0.2 mg every 6 to 8 hours, but patients need to be closely monitored.

- An EPL, incomplete, or missed abortion less than 13 weeks can be managed with misoprostol 800 mcg vaginally.
  - The dose of misoprostol may be repeated in 1 week if evacuation has not occurred.
- Incomplete abortions greater than13 weeks' gestation require surgical intervention with dilation and curettage.
- Any retained products of conception should be managed surgically as well.
- Women who are undergoing expectant/medical management must be counseled on the bleeding and cramping that will likely occur with specific instructions on when to notify the provider if the bleeding becomes excessive.
- Follow-up of patients includes transvaginal ultrasound imaging in 7 to 14 days to confirm passage of tissue.
- Serial beta-HCGs can be used to monitor gradual decline.

CLINICAL PEARL: It is always advisable to assess the entire clinical picture before definitively diagnosing EPL.

REFERENCES

1. American College of Obstetricians and Gynecologists. Practice bulletin no. 200. Early pregnancy loss. https://www.acog.org/Clinical-Guidance-and-Publications/Practice-Bulletins/Committee-on-Practice-Bulletins-Gynecology/Early-Pregnancy-Loss. Published August 29, 2018.
2. Doubilet PM, Benson CB, Bourne T, Blaivas M. Diagnostic criteria for nonviable pregnancy early in the first trimester. *N Engl J Med.* 2013;369:1443–1451. doi:10.1056/NEJMra1302417

ECLAMPSIA

Etiology
- Eclampsia is a complication of preeclampsia with severe features.

Epidemiology[1]
- Eclampsia occurs in about 3% of pregnancies.
- About 20% of patients will be diagnosed between 20 and 30 weeks' gestation, 20% of patients will experience preeclampsia antenatally, and about 20% will present postpartum, usually within the first week.

Clinical Presentation[1,2]

- Patients present with a new-onset grand mal seizure and have a history of preeclampsia.
- Prodromal symptoms include hypertension; frontal, occipital, or thunder-clap headache; visual disturbances, including blurred vision, visual field defects, and homonymous hemianopsia; epigastric or right upper quadrant pain; and ankle clonus.
- Fetal findings include fetal bradycardia, fetal tachycardia, and loss of heart rate variability.

Diagnosis[1,2]

- Gravid women with a history of preeclampsia who present with a tonic–clonic seizure, with no persistent neurological deficit, do not require any further neurological evaluation.

Management[1,2]

- Expeditious management includes prevention of maternal hypoxia with oxygen 8 to 10 L via nonrebreather; prevention of physical trauma with adequate bed rail padding; treatment of severe hypertension, if present; and prevention of recurring seizures with magnesium sulfate.
- Decreased respirations (<12/min) and oliguria (<100 mL/4 hours) are also signs of hypermagnesemia.
- Refractory seizures should be treated with diazepam 5 to 10 mg intravenously or midazolam 1 to 2 mg bolus intravenously.
- The decision to perform a cesarean delivery versus expectant management depends on the gestational age, Bishop score, presentation of the fetus, condition of the mother, and condition of the fetus.

> **CLINICAL PEARL:** In patients receiving magnesium sulfate, patellar reflexes should be tested as a physical manifestation of clinically significant hypermagnesemia includes loss of deep tendon reflexes.

REFERENCES

1. American College of Obstetricians and Gynecologists Task Force on Hypertension in Pregnancy. *Hypertension in Pregnancy*. Washington, DC: Author; 2015.
2. Norwitz ER. Eclampsia. In: Lockwood CJ, Schachter SC, eds. *UptoDate*. https://www.uptodate.com/contents/eclampsia. Updated April 8, 2019.

ECTOPIC PREGNANCY

Etiology

- Most ectopic pregnancies occur in the fallopian tube. Heterotopic pregnancies are ectopic pregnancies that occur in patients with a concurrent intrauterine pregnancy.
- Most patients with ectopic pregnancies do not have the classic risk factors, including prior ectopic pregnancy, history of fallopian tubal damage, pregnancy achieved through assisted reproductive technologies, and prior pelvic surgery.
- Although intrauterine systems decrease the overall risk of ectopic pregnancy, over half of pregnancies in women with an intrauterine system (IUS) are ectopic.[1]

Epidemiology

- Ectopic pregnancies occur in about 2% of all pregnancies.[1]
- Ruptured ectopic pregnancies are a leading source of maternal hemorrhage and death.

Clinical Presentation

- Most often, women will present with early first-trimester vaginal bleeding.
- Pelvic pain may be present.
- In women who present with hemodynamic instability and an acute abdomen, a ruptured ectopic pregnancy must be considered.

Diagnosis

- The diagnosis of ectopic pregnancy requires a menstrual history, a quantitative beta-HCG, and transvaginal ultrasound.
- Careful correlation between the beta-HCG and gestational age must be made.
- Most IUPs are visualized by 5 to 6 weeks' gestation.
- An absent gestational sac with a quantitative beta-HCG above the discriminatory level (up to 3,500 mIU/mL) is considered a nonviable pregnancy, and in up to 70% of patients, an ectopic pregnancy will be diagnosed.[1]
- When there is suspicion of an ectopic pregnancy not confirmed on ultrasound, a repeat quantitative HCG should be drawn in 48 hours.

Management[1]

- Management strategies depend on several criteria.
- Medical management with methotrexate (MTX) can be offered to women if they are hemodynamically stable, have an unruptured mass smaller than 4 cm, and have no contraindications to MTX (Box 3.2).

Box 3.2 Contraindications to Methotrexate in Ectopic Pregnancy

Hemodynamically unstable
A ruptured ectopic pregnancy
An intrauterine pregnancy
Currently breastfeeding
Moderate to severe anemia
Hepatic dysfunction
Renal dysfunction
Immunodeficiency
Sensitivity to methotrexate
Mass >4 cm

- Contraindications to medical management with MTX include an intrauterine pregnancy, a ruptured ectopic pregnancy, current breastfeeding, moderate to severe anemia, hepatic or renal dysfunction, immunodeficiency, and sensitivity to MTX.
- There are various MTX protocols endorsed by ACOG (Figures 3.1 and 3.2).

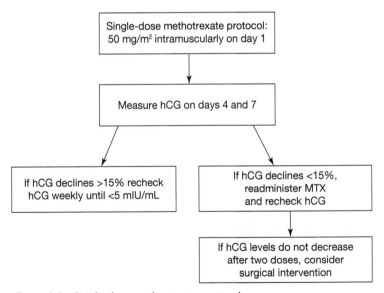

Single-dose methotrexate protocol:
50 mg/m² intramuscularly on day 1

Measure hCG on days 4 and 7

If hCG declines >15% recheck hCG weekly until <5 mIU/mL

If hCG declines <15%, readminister MTX and recheck hCG

If hCG levels do not decrease after two doses, consider surgical intervention

FIGURE **3.1** Single-dose methotrexate protocol.
HCG, human chorionic gonadotropin; MTX, methotrexate.

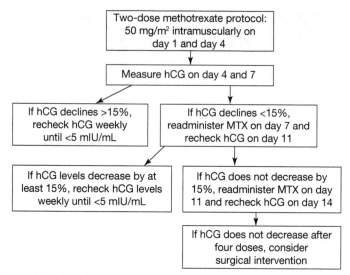

Figure 3.2   Two-dose methotrexate protocol.

HCG, human chorionic gonadotropin; MTX, methotrexate.

- The management of a ruptured ectopic pregnancy is discussed in the section "Ruptured Ectopic Pregnancy" in Chapter 6 Urgent Management of OB/GYN Conditions.

> **Clinical Pearl:** All patients with a positive pregnancy test who present with abnormal vaginal bleeding and/or pelvic pain in the first trimester are considered to have an ectopic pregnancy until proven otherwise.

Reference

1. American College of Obstetricians and Gynecologists. Practice bulletin no. 193. Tubal ectopic pregnancy. https://www.acog.org/Clinical-Guidance-and-Publications/Practice-Bulletins/Committee-on-Practice-Bulletins-Gynecology/Tubal-Ectopic-Pregnancy. Published March 2018.

Gestational Diabetes Mellitus

Etiology[1]

- Insulin resistance during pregnancy is a normal process. The onset of insulin resistance begins in the second trimester and usually peaks during the third trimester.

- The pathophysiology of gestational diabetes is due to maternal pancreatic function that cannot surmount the physiologic insulin resistance of pregnancy.
- Some of the complications associated with gestational diabetes mellitus (GDM) include preeclampsia, macrosomia/large for gestational age, maternal and neonatal birth trauma, hydramnios, and neonatal complications such as hypoglycemia.
- Gravid patients who experience sustained hyperglycemia during organogenesis are at risk for congenital abnormalities.
- Risk factors for GDM include obesity, prior history of GDM, metabolic syndrome, multiple gestation, history of fetal macrosomia, polycystic ovarian syndrome (PCOS), chronic hypertension, sedentarism, ethnicity, and maternal age older than 25 years.

Epidemiology[1,2]

- In the United States, 7% of gravid women will have diabetes, and about 85% of these patients will have GDM
- Certain ethnic groups are at greater risk for developing gestational diabetes, such as Native Americans, African Americans, Hispanics, Southeastern Asians, and Pacific Islanders.
- Women who are diagnosed with GDM are at risk for developing type 1 and type 2 diabetes within 10 years of the pregnancy.

Clinical Presentation

- Most patients are asymptomatic and will be identified with a glucose challenge test (see "Diagnosis" section).

Diagnosis[1]

- Women with risk factors such as obesity and a history of GDM, should be screened at the first prenatal visit.
- If women do not have abnormal glucose levels at the initial prenatal visit, rescreening at 24 to 28 weeks is still recommended.
- Gravid women can be screened using a one-step or two-step approach.
- The one-step approach utilizes a 75-g, 2-hour glucose tolerance test.
- Positive tests from the one-step approach are fasting glucose ≥92 mg/dL, 1 hour ≥180 mg/dL, and 2 hour ≥153 mg/dL. The two-step approach utilizes a 50-g, 1-hour glucose challenge test.
- Positive tests from a 1-hour challenge are serum glucose ≥130 mg/dL to 140 mg/dL, depending on the institution.
- If patients have an elevated glucose, they will undergo a 3-hour glucose tolerance test with 100 g of glucose.
- There is little consensus regarding the glucose-level cutoffs to diagnose gestational diabetes.
- The three guidelines used in the United States are offered by Carpenter and Coustan, the National Diabetes Data Group, and the American Diabetes

TABLE 3.1 Recommended Glucose Thresholds for GDM, mg/dL, 3-Hour OGTT

	Fasting Glucose (mg/dL)	1 Hour Postglucola (mg/dL)	2 Hours Postglucola (mg/dL)	3 Hours Postglucola (mg/dL)
American Diabetes Association	95	180	155	140
Carpenter & Coustan	95	180	155	140
National Diabetes Data Group	105	190	165	145

GDM, gestational diabetes mellitus; OGTT, oral glucose tolerance test.

Source: American College of Obstetricians and Gynecologists. Practice bulletin no. 190. Interim update: gestational diabetes mellitus. https://www.acog.org/Clinical-Guidance-and-Publications/Practice-Bulletins/Committee-on-Practice-Bulletins-Obstetrics/Gestational-Diabetes-Mellitus#1. Published February 2018.

Association. An elevation of at least two glucose levels is required for the diagnosis of GDM (Table 3.1).

- Obstetrician-gynecologist practices will choose which guideline to follow, depending on the overall patient population.
- Gestational diabetes that is controlled with diet and exercise is termed *A1GDM.*
- Gestational diabetes that is controlled with medications is termed *A2GDM.*

Management[1]

- Patients should be offered nutritional counseling with a registered dietician.
- Lifestyle changes, including change in diet and regular exercise, can often result in normoglycemia.
- Glucose targets are as follows:
  - Fasting blood glucose: <95 mg/dL (5.3 mmol/L)
  - 1-hour postprandial blood glucose: <140 mg/dL (7.8 mmol/L)
  - 2-hour postprandial glucose: <120 mg/dL (6.7 mmol/L)
- Patients who are unable to achieve blood glucose levels that fall within the normal range despite lifestyle interventions should begin insulin.
- Metformin is not the first-line medication option unless the patient has such strong objections to using insulin that she would refuse treatment.
- A usual starting dose of insulin is 0.7 to 1.0 units/kg/d.
  - A combination of long-acting, intermediate-acting, and short-acting insulins are used, depending on the patient's glucose profile throughout the day.
- Patients with GDM should begin antepartum fetal surveillance at 32 weeks, including kick counts and nonstress tests (NSTs).
- Patients with A2GDM should be delivered between 39w0d and 39w6d.

- Patients with fetal weight greater than 4,500 g should be offered counseling on the risks and benefits of a scheduled cesarean delivery.
- Patients should be screened for persisting hyperglycemia at the postpartum visit (between 4 and 12 weeks).
  - If abnormal glucose testing persists, that is, fasting glucose greater than or equal to 125 mg/dL or 2-hour oral glucose tolerance test (OGTT) greater than or equl to 199 mg/dL, the patient should be referred for diabetic treatment and counseling.
  - If fasting blood glucose is less than 100 mg/dL or 2-hour OGTT is less than 140 mg/dL, the patient should be screened every 1 to 3 years for type 2 diabetes mellitus (DM).
  - If the patient's fasting glucose is between 100 mg/dL and 124 mg/dL or 2-hour OGTT is 140mg/dL to 199 mg/dL, refer to primary care for impaired glucose tolerance.

> **CLINICAL PEARL:** Patient education is critical when managing a patient with gestational diabetes. Be able to provide appropriate patient education in both written and verbal forms.

REFERENCES

1. American College of Obstetricians and Gynecologists. Practice bulletin no. 190. Interim update: gestational diabetes mellitus. https://www.acog.org/Clinical-Guidance-and-Publications/Practice-Bulletins/Committee-on-Practice-Bulletins-Obstetrics/Gestational-Diabetes-Mellitus#1. Published February 2018.
2. Correa A, Bardenheier B, Elixhauser A, et al. Trends in prevalence of diabetes among delivery hospitalizations, United States, 1993–2009. *Matern Child Health J.* 2015;19:635–642. doi:10.1007/s10995-014-1553-5

GESTATIONAL HYPERTENSION (FORMERLY KNOWN AS PREGNANCY-INDUCED HYPERTENSION)

Etiology

- The pathophysiology of gestational hypertension is currently unknown.

Epidemiology

- Gestational hypertension is the most common cause of hypertension in the gravid patient.
- Women with a history of preeclampsia, overweight/obesity, and multiple-gestation pregnancies are at greater risk of developing gestational hypertension.

Clinical Presentation

- Patients are almost always asymptomatic.

Diagnosis[1,2]

- Diagnosis is defined by new-onset hypertension (systolic blood pressure [BP] ≥140 mmHg and/or diastolic BP ≥90 mmHg) at ≥20 weeks' gestation in a previously normotensive woman and in the absence of proteinuria or new signs of end-organ dysfunction.
- If the BP is ≥140 mmHg and/or diastolic BP ≥90 mmHg, but <160 mmHg systolic and/or 110 mmHg diastolic, BP readings should be documented on at least two occasions at least 4 hours apart.
- Gestational hypertension is considered severe when systolic BP is ≥160 mmHg and/or diastolic BP is ≥110 mmHg.
- Gestational hypertension can be differentiated from preeclampsia if there is no proteinuria, platelet dysfunction (platelets <100,000 cells per microliter), renal dysfunction (serum creatinine >1.1 mg/dL) or doubling of liver transaminases.

Management

- Up to 50% of patients with gestational hypertension develop preeclampsia, so patients must be monitored closely.[1]
- Low-dose aspirin has been recommended to help decrease the risk of preeclampsia.[3]
- Low-dose aspirin can begin at 12 weeks' gestation in women who are considered at risk for developing preeclampsia.
- Women with BPs lower than 160/105 mmHg are generally not treated with antihypertensive therapy but should have twice-weekly BP and urine protein checks. In addition, patients should monitor fetal movements daily.[1]
- Some patients may have NSTs and serial ultrasounds to assess fetal health.
- Women with BPs greater than or equal to 160/110 mmHg should be managed with antihypertensive therapies, such as intravenous labetalol or hydralazine, and delivery considered for patients >34 weeks.[1]
- Most obstetricians will initiate antihypertensive therapy when the diastolic is ≥105 mmHg
  ○ Recommended antihypertensives in pregnancy include labetalol, nifedipine, hydralazine, and methyldopa.
- A course of betamethasone with close monitoring of fetal health is indicated for patients at fewer than 34 weeks' gestation.
- All patients with a hypertensive disorder during pregnancy should have a BP check at 72 hours' postpartum and again at 7 to 10 days' postpartum as preeclampsia and eclampsia can develop during the postpartum period.
- Most women will become normotensive within 12 weeks' postpartum.
- If BP continues to be elevated beyond 12 weeks' postpartum, patients are considered to have chronic hypertension.

> **CLINICAL PEARL:** Patients who are diagnosed with gestational hypertension must be counseled on the signs and symptoms of preeclampsia and advised to report any changes immediately. In addition, you may want to see the patient at shorter intervals between appointments.

REFERENCES

1. American College of Obstetricians and Gynecologists. Task Force on Hypertension in Pregnancy. *Hypertension in Pregnancy.* Washington, DC: Author; 2015.
2. Norwitz ER. In: Lockwood CJ, Schachter SC, eds. Eclampsia. *UptoDate.* https://www.uptodate.com/contents/eclampsia. Updated April 8, 2019.
3. American College of Obstetricians and Gynecologists. Low-dose aspirin use during pregnancy. *Obstet Gynecol.* 2018; 132(1):e44–e52. https://www.acog.org/-/media/Committee-Opinions/Committee-on-Obstetric-Practice/co743.pdf?dmc=1&ts=20190710T1542276868

GESTATIONAL TROPHOBLASTIC DISEASE (MOLAR PREGNANCY/HYDATIDIFORM MOLE)

Etiology

- The etiology of a molar pregnancy depends on whether it is a partial or complete mole (Table 3.2).
- Partial moles are commonly 69,XXX or 69,XXY.
- Complete moles are commonly 46,XX or 46,XY.

Epidemiology[1]

- Gestational trophoblastic disease (GTD) occurs in up to one in 1,500 pregnancies.

TABLE 3.2 Types of Molar Pregnancies

Type of Mole	Fetus	Uterine Size	Theca Lutein Cysts	Malignant Sequalae
Partial mole	Can be present	Small for gestational age	Rare	<5%
Complete mole	Absent	Large for gestational age	Up to 25%	Up to 30%

Source: American College of Obstetricians and Gynecologists. Practice bulletin no. 53. Diagnosis and treatment of gestational trophoblastic disease. acog.org. https://www.acog.org/Clinical-Guidance-and-Publications/Practice -Bulletins/Committee-on-Practice-Bulletins-Gynecology/Diagnosis-and-Treatment-of-Gestational-Trophoblastic -Disease. Reaffirmed 2016.

- In patients with complete moles, up to 30% become malignant.
- Patients with a history of a complete mole or partial mole have a 10-fold risk of developing a subsequent molar pregnancy.

Clinical Presentation[1]

- Patients with complete moles can present with abnormal vaginal bleeding, high HCG levels, hyperemesis, gestational hypertension or preeclampsia prior to 20 weeks' gestation, anemia, hyperthyroidism, coagulopathy, and a uterus that is larger than expected for gestational age.
- Ultrasonography is the cornerstone of diagnosis and will show atypical findings, such as an intrauterine mass with mixed echogenicity and multiple ovarian theca lutein cysts. Adnexa can be enlarged up to 6 cm.
- Patients with partial moles will usually present as a missed abortion.

Diagnosis

- Complete moles are visualized with ultrasonography.
- The classic finding is an intrauterine mass with mixed echogenicity. A Swiss cheese or snowstorm appearance has also been used to describe the findings of a molar pregnancy (Figure 3.3).
- Partial moles are often diagnosed after a missed abortion.

Management[1]

- Surgical evacuation via dilation and curettage of molar pregnancy is necessary.
- Strong consideration should be given for a chest x-ray to evaluate for metastases.
- Laboratory tests include a CBC with platelets, clotting function, blood urea nitrogen (BUN)/creatinine, liver enzymes, bloody type and antibody screen, and HCG.

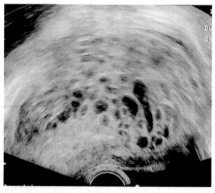

Figure 3.3 Transvaginal ultrasonography showing a molar pregnancy. The pattern is described as a Swiss cheese or snowstorm pattern.
Source: Courtesy of Mikael Häggström.

- Patients should have weekly HCG tests after evacuation until levels drop, then monthly for 6 months.
  - ○ Any increase or plateau in HCG should prompt a careful reevaluation of the patient for malignant postmolar gestational trophoblastic disease.
- Medical management includes weekly prophylactic chemotherapy with intramuscular methotrexate 30mg/m^2 to 50 mg/m^2.[1]
- It is important for women to use reliable contraception while undergoing treatment.
- The management of gestational neoplastic disease is not discussed here.

> **CLINICAL PEARL:** A patient who presents in her first trimester with signs and symptoms of preeclampsia is considered to have a molar pregnancy until proven otherwise.

REFERENCE

1. American College of Obstetricians and Gynecologists. Diagnosis and treatment of gestational trophoblastic disease. ACOG practice bulletin no. 53. https://www.gynecologiconcology-online.net/article/S0090-8258(04)00325-7/pdf

GROUP B STREPTOCOCCAL COLONIZATION

Etiology
- Also known as *Streptococcus agalactiae*
- Colonization of group B *Streptococcus* (GBS) is nonpathogenic to women but can cause severe disease in the newborn
- GBS is responsible for most infectious morbidity and mortality in neonates

Epidemiology[1]
- Up to 30% of gravid patients will be positive for GBS.

Clinical Presentation
- Patients with GBS are asymptomatic.

Diagnosis
- Diagnosis is confirmed via rectovaginal swab testing and culture at 35 to 37 weeks' gestation.
- If a patient has greater than or equal to 10^4 colony-forming units (CFU) of GBS in the urine, the specimen is reported as positive.
- It is not necessary to perform a rectovaginal swab in women with GBS bacteriuria in their current pregnancy.

- If women have a history of a prior delivery of a newborn with GBS disease, she does not need rectovaginal cultures during the current pregnancy as she will receive intrapartum antibiotics anyway

Management[1]

- It is important to provide patient education and to advise the patient of her positive GBS status.
- Patients who are GBS positive should receive intrapartum antibiotics unless rupture of membranes has not yet occurred and a cesarean delivery is planned/performed.
- Patients with a history of delivering a positive GBS neonate will receive intrapartum antibiotics.
- In women who present with preterm labor with preterm rupture of membranes, intrapartum antibiotics will be given if their GBS status is unknown.
- If a woman presents in labor with an unknown GBS status and is at risk of imminent delivery, intrapartum antibiotics are warranted.
- If a woman presents in labor with an unknown GBS status and is febrile ($\geq$100.4°F, $\geq$38°C), intrapartum antibiotics are warranted.
- Intravenous penicillin is the antimicrobial of choice unless the patient has a true immunoglobulin E (IgE)-mediated response. See Figures 3.4 and 3.5 for a summary of treatments of GBS.
- All patients should continue intravenous antibiotics until delivery.

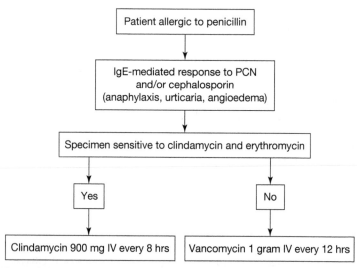

Figure 3.4 Treatment algorithm of GBS in PCN-allergic patients.

GBS, group B *Streptococcus*; IGE, immunoglubulin E; IV, intravenous; PCN, penicillin.

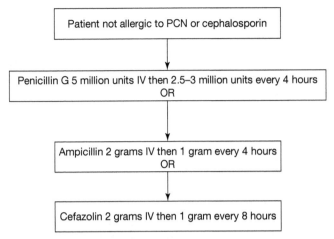

FIGURE 3.5   Treatment of GBS in non-PCN-allergic patient.
GBS, group B *Streptococcus*; IV, intravenous; PCN, penicillin

CLINICAL PEARL: Patient education on the importance of receiving antibiotics during labor is imperative.

REFERENCE

1. American College of Obstetricians and Gynecologists. ACOG practice bulletin no. 782. Prevention of early-onset group B streptococcal disease in newborns. https://www.acog.org/Clinical-Guidance-and-Publications/Committee-Opinions/ Committee-on-Obstetric-Practice/Prevention-of-Early-Onset-Group-B -Streptococcal-Disease-in-Newborns#here. Published June 25, 2019.

HELL P SYNDROME[1]

Etiology

- HELLP stands for *hemolysis, elevated liver enzymes,* and *low platelets.*
- The pathophysiology of HELLP is poorly understood.
- HELLP may originate from abnormal placental development resulting in coagulopathy and hepatic inflammation.
- Patients at risk for developing HELLP include patients with a prior history of preeclampsia or HELLP, advanced maternal age, and European ancestry.

Epidemiology[1]

- Some research indicates HELLP may be a severe form of preeclampsia, but up to 20% of patients will not have antecedent hypertension or proteinuria.
- Approximately 0.2% of pregnancies overall and up to 20% of women with severe preeclampsia/eclampsia will develop HELLP.

Clinical Presentation

- Gravid patients may present with fatigue/malaise, midepigastric or right upper quadrant pain, nausea and/or emesis, and an elevated BP with proteinuria.
- AST and lactate dehydrogenase (LDH) are markedly elevated.

Diagnosis[1]

- Diagnosis is based on laboratory analysis.
- Anemia will be present with schistocytes (also called *helmet cells*) on peripheral smear; hemolysis may also present with elevated indirect bilirubin level and low serum haptoglobin concentration.
- Platelets will be less than 100,000 cells per microliter.
- Total bilirubin will be greater than or equal to 1.2 mg/dL, and hemolysis results in an increase in indirect bilirubin as well.
- AST will be at least twice the upper limit of normal.
- Elevated BUN and creatinine can occur in renal failure.
- Fibrinogen will be decreased due to the coagulopathy, whereas D-dimer will be increased secondary to fibrinolysis.

Management[1]

- The management of patients with HELLP is similar to that of patients with preeclampsia with severe features.
- Gestations less than 34 weeks are treated with magnesium sulfate and antihypertensives as indicated.
- The use of corticosteroids in HELLP for gestational age less than 34 weeks is disputed, but most physicians will administer one course.
- Dexamethasone has been shown to moderately increase platelets over betamethasone.
- To prevent maternal deterioration and/or fetal demise, expectant management usually does not last more than 48 hours.
- Gestations longer than 34 weeks should be delivered as delivery is curative.
- Patients with HELLP are at risk for developing DIC, placental abruption, acute renal failure, and acute pulmonary edema. Therefore, patients must be managed quickly and carefully, and often in consultation with maternal–fetal medicine specialists.

CLINICAL PEARL: If you suspect HELLP, act expeditiously by ordering labs STAT.

REFERENCE

1. Sibai BM. HELLP syndrome. In: Lockwood CJ, Lindor KD, eds. *UptoDate*. https://www.uptodate.com/contents/hellp-syndrome. Updated August 1, 2019.

HERPES INFECTION IN PREGNANCY

Etiology
- Genital herpes is caused by the herpes simplex virus (HSV). Most cases are HSV-2.
- Pregnant patients can present with an initial outbreak or a recurrent outbreak during pregnancy.

Epidemiology[1]
- About 22% of pregnant women have a history of genital herpes.
- Two percent of pregnant patients will have their initial outbreak during pregnancy.
- Approximately 30% of pregnant patients will have HSV-2 antibodies.
- Up to 2,000 infants are born with neonatal HSV infections.
- Women with genital herpes are at risk for preterm delivery.

Clinical Presentation
- Patients may report a vulvar sore, vulvar or vaginal pain, and pruritus.
- The lesions of genital herpes are painful ulcerations or vesicles.
- The vulva is most often affected but cervical lesions can sometimes be visualized.
- In women with vulvar lesions, there can be significant erythema and edema present.
- Sometimes patients will experience vaginal discharge and dysuria as well.

Diagnosis
- Diagnosis can be made based on physical examination.
- Diagnosis is confirmed with culture or viral polymerase chain reaction (PCR) testing.
- An older test was the Tzanck smear, is not used in the United States due to its poor sensitivity and specificity and availability of more sensitive and specific testing.

Management[1]
- Antiviral medications are the mainstay of pharmacologic management (Table 3.3).
- The Centers for Disease Control and Prevention (CDC) has various approved antiviral regimens, depending on whether the patient has an initial outbreak, a recurrent outbreak, or is being treated for chronic suppression.

TABLE 3.3 Overview of the Pharmacologic Management of Genital Herpes in Pregnancy

First-Line Treatment	Alternative
Initial outbreak	
Acyclovir 400 mg three times a day for 7–10 days	Valacyclovir 1,000 mg twice a day for 7–10 days
Recurrent outbreaks	
Acyclovir 400 mg three times a day for 5 days OR 800 mg twice a day for 5 days	Valacyclovir 500 mg twice a day for 3 days OR 1,000 mg daily for 5 days
Chronic suppression	
Acyclovir 400 mg three times a day starting at 36 weeks until delivery	Valacyclovir 500 mg twice a day starting at 36 weeks until delivery

- Shedding of HSV can last up to 2 weeks, including during the prodromal stage. Thus, patient education is essential.
- It is essential to prevent transmission to the fetus, so suppressive therapy with daily antivirals should begin at 36 weeks.
- A patient with a current outbreak at the time of delivery should have a cesarean.
- It is best to perform the cesarean within 4 to 6 hours of rupture of membranes.

CLINICAL PEARL: It is not clinically relevant to determine whether the genital HSV is type 1 or 2 because the management is the same.

REFERENCE

1. Grove MK. Genital herpes in pregnancy. In: Ramus RM, ed. *Medscape.* https://emedicine.medscape.com/article/274874-overview#a1. Updated January 20, 2017.

HYPEREMESIS GRAVIDARUM

Etiology

- The etiology of hyperemesis gravidarum (HG) is poorly understood.
- Some of the theories of HG include a hormonally mediated psychologic propensity as well as an evolutionary adaptation.
- HG is a severe form of nausea and vomiting in pregnancy.
- Treatment of nausea and vomiting may prevent progression to HG.

Epidemiology[1]

- Prevalence rates of nausea and vomiting in pregnancy are around 80%.
- Incidence of HG can vary; it occurs inup to 3% of pregnancies.
- Incidence rates of HG vary due to a lack of specific diagnostic criteria.

Clinical Presentation

- Patients with HG will present with recurrent, unremitting nausea and vomiting.
- In a severe form of HG, patients may present with neurological manifestations of Wernicke's (thiamine-deficiency) encephalopathy.
- In its most severe form, HG can also result in esophageal rupture, pneumothorax, and acute tubular necrosis.

Diagnosis

- Diagnosis is usually made by history, but several physical exam findings support the diagnosis.
- Patients who present after 9 weeks' gestation should be ruled out for other disorders, including gastroparesis, pancreatitis, hepatitis, diabetic ketoacidosis, hyperthyroidism, idiopathic intracranial hypertension, vestibular or central nervous system (CNS) lesions, and acute fatty liver of pregnancy.
- It is important to rule out other disorders of pregnancy that can result in HG, including molar pregnancy and multiple gestation.
- A thorough history and physical examination should be done on all patients with HG.
- Ketonuria and at least a 5% weight loss from prepregnancy levels are often used to substantiate the diagnosis.

Management[1]

- No specific dietary changes have been shown to reduce HG.
- Over-the-counter ginger products may relieve mild symptoms.
- Other nonpharmacologic treatments that have been used with variable success include acupressure, acupuncture, and wrist electrical nerve stimulation.
- The pharmacologic management of HG includes the following:
  - Vitamin B6 (pyridoxine) 10 to 25 mg three to four times a day
  - Doxylamine 12.5 mg three to four times a day
  - Vitamin B6 10 mg with doxylamine; 10-mg dose is available as a combination therapy and can be taken three times a day, with two tablets taken at bedtime
  - Vitamin B6 20 mg with doxylamine; 20-mg dose is available as a combination therapy and can be taken twice a day
  - Other over-the-counter pharmacologic options include diphenhydramine and dimenhydrinate, 25–50 mg three to four times a day
  - Other prescription options include metoclopramide, promethazine, chlorpromazine, prochlorperazine, trimethobenzamide, and ondansetron

- ○ Ondansetron 4 mg can be taken every 6 to 8 hours
- ○ Metoclopramide, promethazine, chlorpromazine, and prochlorperazine can cause extrapyramidal side effects as they are dopamine antagonists
  - These medications are sometimes administered with diphenhydramine to help prevent the extrapyramidal side effects
- ○ For severe, refractory HG of at least 3 weeks' duration that requires intravenous fluid administration, thiamine 100 mg should be given with the initial intravenous fluid bolus followed by thiamine 100 mg daily for 3 days with multivitamins
- ○ Methylprednisolone can also be used in severe, refractory HG
- ○ Enteral feedings may need to be considered in patients with persistent, refractory HG accompanied by persistent weight loss

> **CLINICAL PEARL:** HG can be debilitating. Some patients will question whether or not they want to continue with the pregnancy because they feel so awful. Patient education and support are critical when managing these patients.

REFERENCE

1. American College of Obstetricians and Gynecologists. ACOG Practice Bulletin No. 189. Nausea and vomiting of pregnancy. https://www.acog.org/Clinical-Guidance-and-Publications/Practice-Bulletins/Committee-on-Practice-Bulletins-Obstetrics/Nausea-and-Vomiting-of-Pregnancy. Published January 2018.

INTRAUTERINE GROWTH RESTRICTION

Etiology[1]

- The etiology of IUGR can be divided into fetal, placental, and maternal issues.
- Fetal issues include the trisomies and gastroschisis.
- Placental issues include abnormal placentation.
- Maternal issues include comorbid conditions such as diabetes, hypertensive disorder, and autoimmune disease.
  - ○ Other issues include substance use, fetotoxic exposures to medications, and infections such as cytomegalovirus, rubella, and syphilis.

Epidemiology

- The actual incidence and prevalence of IUGR is not apparent as there has been little consensus on the definition of IUGR.

- Women who have delivered small-for-gestational-age babies should be screened for IUGR in subsequent pregnancies.

Clinical Presentation

- Providers may be alerted to a possibility of IUGR if the fundal height measurements are less than expected for gestational age, particularly in women at risk for developing IUGR.

Diagnosis

- The diagnosis is confirmed with ultrasound.
- ACOG recommends that in fetuses who have an estimated fetal weight less than the 10th percentile, a diagnosis of IUGR can be made.

Management[1]

- IUGR fetuses should have repeat ultrasounds every 3 to 4 weeks.
- Umbilical artery Doppler velocimetry is recommended to evaluate the presence or progression of uteroplacental insufficiency.
- NST with or without a biophysical profile is also indicated, usually beginning at 32 weeks.
- Timing of delivery of an IUGR fetus depends on several issues, including the presence of oligohydramnios, abnormal uterine artery Doppler velocimetry, and other comorbidities.

> **CLINICAL PEARL:** IUGR should not be diagnosed by one solitary measurement. Look at the entire clinical picture and obtain serial measurements if the concern continues.

REFERENCE

1. American College of Obstetricians and Gynecologists. ACOG practice bulletin no. 204. Interim update: Fetal growth restriction. https://www.acog.org/Clinical%20Guidance%20and%20Publications/Practice%20Bulletins/Committee%20on%20Practice%20Bulletins%20Obstetrics/Fetal%20Growth%20Restriction.aspx#box1. Published January 24, 2019.

LACTATIONAL MASTITIS

Etiology

- Lactational mastitis occurs in breastfeeding women.
- Lactational mastitis can occur when there are problems with engorgement or proper drainage.
- Milk duct blockages, infrequent feeding, maternal stress, and nipple excoriations can cause mastitis.

- The most common bacterial etiology of mastitis is *Staphylococcus aureus*.
- Cases of methicillin-resistant *Staphylococcus aureus* (MRSA) are occurring more frequently.
- Less common bacterial species are *Streptococcus pyogenes* (group A or B), *Escherichia coli*, *Bacteroides* species, *Corynebacterium*.

Epidemiology[1]

- Lactational mastitis can occur in up to 10% of breastfeeding women.

Clinical Presentation

- The patient will present with a painful, erythematous, and swollen breast.
- Many women will also have fever, chills, myalgias, and fatigue.

Diagnosis

- Diagnosis is based on history and physical examination.
- No cultures or other laboratory or imaging are necessary.
  - ○ However, lactational mastitis must be differentiated from a breast abscess, which is a complication of untreated mastitis.
- An abscess will have an area of tender fluctuance; breast ultrasonography can help differentiate between the two if there is any confusion

Management[1]

- The management consists of appropriate antimicrobial therapy combined with complete breast emptying and nonsteroidal anti-inflammatory drugs (NSAIDs) for pain (Table 3.4).
- In most cases, patients should be encouraged to continue breastfeeding.

TABLE 3.4 Pharmacologic Treatment of Lactational Mastitis

Type of Lactational Mastitis	Drugs of Choice	Notes
Uncomplicated	Dicloxacillin 500 mg four times a day for 10 days OR Cephelexin 500 mg four times a day for 10 days	If PCN-allergic, may use clarithromycin 500 mg twice daily for 10–14 days OR clindamycin 300 mg three times a day for 10–14 days
Complicated or MRSA suspected	Clindamycin 300 mg three times a day for 10–14 days OR trimethoprim/sulfamethoxazole DS twice a day for 10 days	Trimethoprim/sulfamethoxazole should be used after the first month postpartum
Severe infection, worsening infection despite antibiotics	Vancomycin 15–20 mg/kg/dose every 8 hours (maximum dose 2 g/dose)	Patients should be monitored closely for sepsis

DS, double strength; MRSA, methicillin-resistant *Staphylococcus aureus*; PCN, penicillin.

- Dicloxacillin or cephalexin 500 mg QID for 10 days is the recommended first-line antimicrobial choice.
- Clindamycin 300 mg three times a day is an appropriate alternative for uncomplicated lactational mastitis and suspected or confirmed MRSA.
- Another option for MRSA is trimethoprim/sulfamethoxazole double strength one tablet twice a day for 10 days, but only after the first month postpartum.
- Patients with severe infection, particularly if hemodynamically compromised or worsening despite antimicrobial therapy, should be given vancomycin 15 to 20 mg/kg/dose every 8 hours with care not to exceed 2 g per dose.

CLINICAL PEARL: A patient who does not respond to antimicrobial therapy should be assessed for possible MRSA and ruled out for inflammatory breast cancer.

REFERENCE

1. Miller AC. Mastitis empiric therapy. In: Herchline TE, ed. *Medscape*. https://emedicine.medscape.com/article/2028354-overview. Updated March 12, 2019.

NORMAL LABOR AND DELIVERY

Etiology
- The role of a laborist is to assist the patient when necessary and be vigilant about situations that require expert intervention.
- The most common morphology of the pelvis is gynecoid (Figure 3.6). This shape allows for the successful passage of the neonate in most labors

Clinical Presentation[1,2]
- Most women in labor will present with complaints of uterine contractions, low-back pain, or possible spontaneous rupture of membranes.
- Normal labor is defined as a progressive dilation and cervical effacement that results from uterine contractions.
- Contractions occur at least every 5 minutes and last at least 30 seconds.
- Labor is divided into three stages:
  - The first stage is divided into latent and active labor.
    - According to Friedman's curve, this stage can take from 6 to 18 hours in a nullipara and 2 to 10 hours in a primipara.

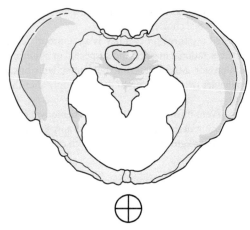

FIGURE 3.6 Schematic illustration of the gynecoid pelvis. This shape is the most common and allows for successful passage of the neonate in most labors.

○ Friedman's curve was once used to define and quantify the duration of latent and active labor. A prolonged latent phase was diagnosed when it exceeded 20 hours in nulliparas and 14 hours in multiparas.

- Latent phase: Progressive cervical dilation and effacement up to 4 cm
  - It is important to document fetal presentation during this phase.
- Active phase: More rapid dilation from 4 to 5 cm until delivery
  - In nulliparas, the cervix usually dilates at about 1 cm per hour, and about 1.2 cm per hour in multiparas.
  - Fetal station is assessed (Figure 3.7). Fetal station is the relationship between the fetal head to the maternal ischial spines. Station is measured by −5 to +5 cm. Zero is at the ischial spines. Crowning is +5 cm, or when the greatest fetal head diameter is at the vulva. Some providers report on a scale of − 3 to +3. When the fetal head is in the pelvic outlet, this is +3.

○ The second stage: Complete dilation that resultants in delivery of the infant.

- Can last minutes to hours. Primiparas can take up to 3 hours, and multiparas usually complete the second stage within 30 minutes.
- Descent of the fetus through the vaginal canal is monitored to ensure progress is appropriate.
- The seven cardinal movements of labor have been used to describe the fetal movements through the vaginal canal. These are referred to as *EDFI triple E*: **e**ngagement, **d**escent, **f**lexion, **i**nternal rotation, **e**xtension, **e**xternal rotation, and **e**xpulsion (Figure 3.8).

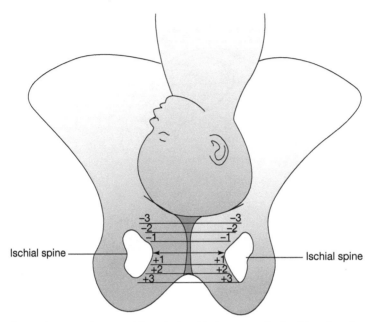

FIGURE **3.7**   Fetal station: The relationship between the fetal head to the maternal ischial spines.

- Extension of the head allows passage beneath the maternal symphysis.
- External rotation of the head after delivery allows facilitation of shoulder delivery.
  ○ The third stage is delivery of the placenta.

Diagnosis
- Normal labor is defined as a progressive dilation and cervical effacement (thinning) that results from uterine contractions.
- Contractions must occur at least every 5 minutes and last at least 30 seconds for active labor.
- Uterine tocodynamometry shows the frequency, duration, and strength of uterine contractions, as well as the fetal heart rate.
- If performing a sterile pelvic speculum exam to assess for rupture of membranes, there may be pooling of amniotic fluid in the posterior aspect of the speculum.
  ○ In addition, a fern test and a nitrazine test may be performed.
  ○ The fern test requires you to collect the fluid from the posterior fornix of the vagina using a sterile swab and placing the fluid on a slide to dry.

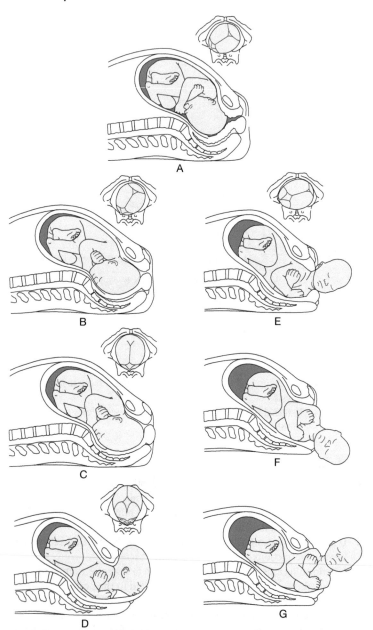

FIGURE 3.8 Seven cardinal movements of labor through the vaginal canal: (A) engagement, (B) descent, (C) flexion, (D) internal rotation, (E) extension, (F) external rotation, and (G) expulsion.

Examination under the microscope may reveal a ferning pattern. This is pathognomonic for amniotic fluid.

○ You may also check the pH of the vaginal fluid with nitrazine paper. Amniotic fluid has a high pH, so if the nitrazine paper turns blue, it may mean that rupture of membranes has occurred. However, nitrazine testing is neither specific nor sensitive and should only be used as an adjunct. Blood, semen, and certain vaginal bacteria may also cause an elevated pH.

Management
- Management depends on each clinical situation and stage of labor.

> **CLINICAL PEARL:** The best way to distinguish Braxton–Hicks (false labor) from actual labor contractions is by assessing the cervix. Braxton–Hicks are not strong enough contractions to dilate and efface the cervix.

REFERENCES

1. Hobel CJ, Zakowski M. Normal labor, delivery, and postpartum care. In: Hacker NF, Gambone JC, Hobel CJ, eds. *Hacker and Moore's Essentials of Obstetrics and Gynecology.* 6th ed. Philadelphia, PA: Saunders/Elsevier; 2016:96–124.
2. American College of Obstetrics and Gynecology. Obstetric care consensus no. 1. Safe prevention of the primary cesarean delivery. *Obstet Gynecol.* 2014;123(3):693–711. doi:10.1097/01.AOG.0000444441.04111.1d

PLACENTA PREVIA

Etiology
- A low-lying placenta occurs when the edge of the placenta is less than 2 cm from, but not covering, the internal os.
- *Placenta previa* is defined as the covering of the internal os by the placenta.
- Risk factors include previous placenta previa, previous cesarean delivery, multiparity, and multiple gestation.

Epidemiology[1,2]
- Placenta previa occurs in about five per 1,000 pregnancies.
- Patients with a history of placenta previa and a previous uterine incision, particularly a cesarean incision, are at risk for developing placenta accreta, placenta increta, and placenta percreta.

Clinical Presentation

- Painless vaginal bleeding in the third trimester is a common sign in a patient with placenta previa.
- A low-lying placenta, or a placenta previa, is usually diagnosed at a second-trimester screening ultrasound.
- Patients who present with second- or third-trimester bleeding should undergo ultrasonographic imaging before a digital exam to rule out a placenta previa.
- Over 90% of second-trimester low-lying placentas will migrate to a superior location by the third trimester.[3]

Diagnosis

- Diagnosis is accomplished with ultrasound imaging.

Management[2]

- Women who are diagnosed with an asymptomatic placental previa should be advised to abstain from sexual intercourse, avoid inserting anything into the vagina, refrain from heavy lifting, or engaging in strenuous exercise.
- Digital vaginal exams should be avoided.
- Asymptomatic patients who are diagnosed in the second trimester should undergo repeat ultrasound imaging at 32 weeks to assess location and presence of coexisting placenta accreta.
  - ○ If the previa still exists, a repeat ultrasound at 36 weeks can be undertaken. If the previa is still present (<2 cm from the internal os), cesarean delivery is scheduled.
- Patients are considered high risk if they have been diagnosed with a low-lying placenta or previa located anteriorly in the area of a prior uterine scar from cesarean delivery.
  - ○ These patients are at significant risk for a placental accreta and hemorrhage so appropriate preoperative hemorrhage precautions must be taken, with experienced personnel who are prepared for an emergency cesarean and possible hysterectomy. Thus, delivery should occur in the surgical suite.
- Management of an actively bleeding placenta previa is similar to the management of abruptio placentae.
- Maternal hemodynamic stabilization is paramount.
- Continuous external fetal heart rate monitoring should be initiated as soon as possible. If any evidence of fetal distress appears despite basic interventions, delivery is indicated.

> **CLINICAL PEARL:** Always check the most recent ultrasound before performing a digital exam on a patient in the third trimester to make sure there is no placenta previa.

REFERENCES

1. Cresswell JA, Ronsmans C, Calvert C, Filippi V. Prevalence of placenta praevia by world region: a systematic review and meta-analysis. *Trop Med Int Health.* 2013;18(6):712–724. doi:10.1111/tmi.12100
2. Wagner SA. Third trimester vaginal bleeding. In: DeCherney AH, Nathan L, Laufer N, Roman AS, eds. *Current Diagnosis and Treatment: Obstetrics and Gynecology.* New York, NY: McGraw-Hill Medical; 2013:310–316.
3. Oyelese Y, Smulian JC. Placenta previa, placenta accreta, and vasa previa. *Obstet Gynecol.* 2006;107(4):927. doi:10.1097/01.AOG.0000207559.15715.98

POSTPARTUM DEPRESSION

Etiology[1,2]

- The etiology and pathophysiology of postpartum depression is poorly understood, but hippocampal responses to hormonal fluctuations have been identified as possible causative factors.
- Women with preexisting depression or a history of depression are at greatest risk of developing postpartum depression. As such, ACOG recommends screening for depression at least once during each pregnancy.
- Severe postpartum depression is associated with impaired newborn bonding, breastfeeding problems, suicide, and infanticide.

Epidemiology[2]

- About 16% of patients will develop postpartum depression.
- The majority of women with postpartum depression experience symptoms in the first month postpartum, but symptoms can occur up to 1 year after delivery.
- Some women will experience depressive symptoms during pregnancy.

Clinical Presentation

- The presentation of postpartum depression is similar to that of major depression.
- It is important to screen for the presence of symptoms as patients may feel embarrassed or afraid to tell a healthcare provider about what they are feeling.

Diagnosis[1]

- Diagnosis requires a careful history. Women who have five or more of the common symptoms of depression that have been present for at least 2 weeks, and at least one of the symptoms is either a depressed mood or a loss of interest, can be diagnosed with postpartum depression.

- Sometimes women with postpartum depression will experience insomnia or hypersomnia, feelings of worthlessness or incompetence, guilt, indecisiveness, agitation, or profound fatigue.
- All women who present with symptoms of postpartum depression must be asked about suicidal or homicidal ideation.
- Postpartum depression can occur any time within the first 12 months following delivery.
- The Edinburgh Postnatal Depression Scale has been validated as a useful screening tool. There are 10 questions, each with three answer options. Thus, the highest score is a 30. A score greater than 10 is suggestive of postpartum depression.

Management[1]

- Mild to moderate postpartum depression should be initially managed with referral to a mental health specialist for cognitive behavioral therapy.
- Patients with a history of depression, history of postpartum depression, and severe postpartum depression should receive pharmacologic therapy and cognitive behavioral therapy.
- Selective serotonin reuptake inhibitors, such as sertraline, citalopram, and escitalopram, are the preferred medications, even if the patient is breastfeeding.
- Research is being conducted on the use of brexanolone, a progesterone metabolite, for the treatment of postpartum depression.

CLINICAL PEARL: Patients with postpartum depression need emotional support and patient education on the expected course and outcome of their disease. It is advisable to have the patient return for a reassessment within 1 or 2 weeks to make sure she is progressing positively.

REFERENCES

1. American College of Obstetrics and Gynecology. Committee opinion no. 757: Interim update: Screening for perinatal depression. acog.org. https://www.acog.org/Clinical-Guidance-and-Publications/Committee-Opinions/Committee-on-Obstetric-Practice/Screening-for-Perinatal-Depression. Published October 24, 2018.
2. Gaillard A, Le Strat Y, Mandelbrot L, et al. Predictors of postpartum depression: prospective study of 264 women followed during pregnancy and postpartum. *Psychiatry Res.* 2014;215(2):341–346. doi:10.1016/j.psychres.2013.10.003

POSTPARTUM HEMORRHAGE

Etiology

- The underlying etiolmanagement includes tranexamicogies of postpartum hemorrhage (PPH) include uterine atony, trauma, retained tissue (such as retained placenta and placenta accreta), and coagulopathies.
- There are several risk factors for the development of PPH. Prolonged use of oxytocin, multiparity (greater than four deliveries), multiple gestation, and fetal macrosomia can cause uterine atony leading to PPH.
- Coagulopathies can occur in preeclamptic patients, those with sepsis, inherited coagulopathies, and who are on anticoagulation for therapeutic purposes.
- A history of a PPH is an additional risk factor for a PPH.

Epidemiology[1]

- PPH is the leading cause of maternal morbidity in the United States, and a leading cause of maternal mortality in the world.

Clinical Presentation

- Often, patients will remain relatively asymptomatic until significant blood loss has occurred.
- Once patients become hypotensive and tachycardic, considerable blood loss has already occurred.
- Blood loss of more than 500 mL for a vaginal delivery or more than 1,000 mL for a cesarean delivery constitutes a hemorrhage, prompting the initiation of a PPH algorithm. However, ACOG recently refined the definition to "cumulative blood loss ≥1,000 mL **or** bleeding associated with signs/symptoms of hypovolemia within 24 hours of the birth process regardless of delivery route".[1]

Diagnosis

- Visual estimates of blood loss are inadequate. Blood loss must be quantified. Under-buttocks calibrated drapes help with quantification, and blood-soaked items should be weighed.

Management [1,2]

- Uterotonics, such as oxytocin, are employed during the third phase of labor to help prevent PPH. This is called the *active management of the third phase of labor (AMTSL)*.
- When PPH occurs, prompt notification of the PPH response team is advised. Prompt treatment of the underlying cause of the hemorrhage, if known, is essential. Therefore, exploration of the vagina and uterus to

assess for trauma, retained tissue, uterine atony or involution, and uterine rupture if the patient is having a vaginal birth after cesarean (VBAC).

- Initiating basic life-support measures is indicated. This includes obtaining intravenous access with two large-bore needles; administering oxygen and isotonic crystalloid solutions; measuring urine output and vital signs; and monitoring hematocrit, electrolytes, and coagulation factors (fibrinogen concentration, PT, activated partial thromboplastin time [aPTT]) are essential.

- Unless the patient has already been typed and crossmatched, order these as well.

- It is also important to keep the patient warm.

- Perform uterine massage when indicated.

- Medical management includes tranexamic acid 1 g, 10 mL of a 100 mg/mL solution, infused over 10 to 20 minutes; oxytocin 40 units in 1 L of normal saline intravenously or 10 units intramuscularly/directly into the myometrium; carboprost 250 mcg intramuscularly every 15 to 90 minutes for a maximum dose of 2 mg or eight doses unless the patient is asthmatic; and methylergonovine 0.2 mg intramuscularly or directly in the myometrium.

- Misoprostol administered sublingually, buccally, and rectally has been used extensively as well. Data show that misoprostol is not superior to other uterotonics, can cause hyperthermia, and can take longer to achieve peak concentrations.

- When patients are hemorrhaging, vaginal administration is not indicated because the drug will not be adequately absorbed.

- Intrauterine tamponades are appropriate for patients with uterine atony and lower segment bleeding.

- Surgical management is appropriate when bleeding continues.

- Transfusion protocols vary by institution. Most patients will receive O negative packed red blood cells and fresh frozen plasma in a one-to-one ratio. If a massive transfusion occurs, it is important to monitor serum calcium and potassium as hypocalcemia and hyperkalemia can occur.

- Massive hemorrhage protocols may also include apheresis platelets, cryoprecipitate, and recombinant activated factor VIIa.

- Uterine artery embolization by an interventional radiologist should be considered prior to surgery if available.

- Surgical management is appropriate when bleeding continues. Cesarean and hysterectomy will cause an additional loss of 2 to 3 L of blood in an already unstable patient, so embolization is preferred. It is associated with less morbidity and blood loss if it can be performed expeditiously.

CLINICAL PEARL: The leading cause of postpartum hemorrhage is uterine atony.

References

1. American College of Obstetricians and Gynecologists. Practice bulletin no. 183. Postpartum hemorrhage. https://www.acog.org/Clinical-Guidance-and -Publications/Practice-Bulletins/Committee-on-Practice-Bulletins-Obstetrics/ Postpartum-Hemorrhage. Published October 2017.
2. World Health Organization. WHO recommendations on prevention and treatment of postpartum haemorrhage and the WOMAN trial. https://www.who.int/ reproductivehealth/topics/maternal_perinatal/pph-woman-trial/en. Published June 15, 2017.

Preeclampsia

Etiology

- Preeclampsia is characterized by new-onset hypertension in a previously normotensive patient with the presence of proteinuria or other end-organ damage, such as elevated liver transaminases, serum creatinine, and platelet dysfunction.
- The pathophysiology is poorly understood, but some theories involve abnormal placental spiral arteriole development, immunologic dysfunction, and placental ischemia.

Epidemiology[1]

- Preclampsia can complicate up to 10% of pregnancies.
- Preeclampsia is a leading cause of maternal and fetal morbidity and mortality.
- Common fetal sequelae include intrauterine growth restriction, small for gestational age, and oligohydramnios.

Clinical Presentation

- Most preeclampsia will manifest after 20 weeks' gestation.
- The presence of preeclampsia prior to 20 weeks' gestation requires a molar pregnancy be ruled out.
- Some patients will be asymptomatic.
- All patients should be asked about the severe symptoms of preeclampsia, such as epigastric or right upper quadrant pain, visual changes, swelling, or headaches.
- Physical examination should include inspection for peripheral edema and auscultation of the chest for pulmonary edema.
- BP higher than 160/110 mmHg is a hypertensive emergency and patients must be managed expeditiously.

TABLE **3.5** Diagnostic Criteria for Preeclampsia

Preeclampsia Without Severe Features	Preeclampsia With Severe Features
BPs >140/90 mmHg on two occasions 4 hours apart OR 160/110 mmHg on one occasion AND Proteinuria >300 mg/24 hours with a urine protein/creatinine ratio >0.3 mg/dL	Platelet count <100,000 cells per microliter Liver transaminase elevation Pulmonary edema Visual or cerebral changes Serum creatinine >1.1 mg/dL OR Doubling of a previous serum creatinine

BP, blood pressure.

Diagnosis[1]

- Preeclampsia is classified as either "without severe features" or "with severe features" (Table 3.5).
- Preeclampsia without severe features is diagnosed with BPs higher than 140/90 mmHg on two occasions 4 hours apart (or 160/110 mmHg on one occasion) AND proteinuria greater than 300 mg/24 hours with a urine protein/creatinine ratio greater than 0.3 mg/dL.
- All patients with new-onset hypertension should have a CBC with platelets, liver transaminases, LDH, creatinine, bilirubin, and uric acid,
- Changes consistent with preeclampsia with severe features include thrombocytopenia, increase in creatinine concentration to more than 1.1 mg/dL, and doubling of hepatic transaminases.
- For the diagnosis of preeclampsia with severe features, quantified proteinuria of more than 5 g in 24 hours is no longer required.
- Platelet count less than 100,000 cells permicroliter, liver transaminase elevation, serum creatinine greater than 1.1 mg/dL (or doubling of a previous serum creatinine), pulmonary edema, and visual or cerebral changes constitute severe features of preeclampsia.

Management[1,2]

- Management algorithms depend on gestational age and presence or absence of severe features.
- Pregnancies at less than 34 weeks' gestation with severe features should be admitted to labor and delivery for continuous fetal monitoring, maternal BP and urine output monitoring, administration of corticosteroids, and laboratory evaluation for renal function and the development of HELLP.
- In patients with BP less than 160/110 mmHg and without severe features, delivery is indicated once the patient reaches 37 weeks.
- Patients with BP higher than 160/110 mmHg should receive intravenous labetalol or hydralazine.
  - ○ Oral nifedipine can be used if no intravenous access is available.
- Magnesium sulfate is neuroprotective.
  - ○ Magnesium sulfate is not an antihypertensive therapy.

- ○ It is administered to women with severe features to help protect against the development of eclampsia but can also be considered for women without severe features.
- ○ The standard is a 4-g loading dose, followed by 1 g/hr.
- Patients at 34w0d and later should be considered for delivery following a course of antenatal corticosteroids (if not already done), or immediate delivery if there is evidence of fetal distress, ruptured membranes, oliguria, serum creatinine level of 1.5 mg/dL or greater, pulmonary edema, HELLP syndrome, eclampsia, platelets less than 100,000 cells per microliter, coagulopathy, and placental abruption.
- ACOG endorses the use of low-dose aspirin for the prevention of preeclampsia in women with a history of preeclampsia or risk factors for the development of preeclampsia (such as multifetal gestation, type 1 or 2 diabetes, chronic hypertension, autoimmune disease, and renal disease).
- Low-dose aspirin can begin at 12 weeks' gestation.[3]

> **CLINICAL PEARL:** In any pregnant patient with new onset hypertension, consider the possibility of preeclampsia and be prepared to evaluate the patient with the appropriate physical examination and laboratory studies.

REFERENCES

1. American College of Obstetricians and Gynecologists. Task Force on Hypertension in Pregnancy. *Hypertension in Pregnancy.* Washington, DC: Author; 2015.
2. Norwitz ER. Eclampsia. In: Lockwood CJ, Schachter SC, eds. *UptoDate.* https://www.uptodate.com/contents/eclampsia. Updated April 8, 2019.
3. American College of Obstetricians and Gynecologists. ACOG Committee Opinion No. 743. Low-dose aspirin use during pregnancy. *Obstet Gynecol.* 2018; 132(1):e44–e52. https://www.acog.org/-/media/Committee-Opinions/Committee-on-Obstetric-Practice/co743.pdf?dmc=1&ts=20190710T1542276868

PRELABOR RUPTURE OF MEMBRANES/PRETERM PRELABOR RUPTURE OF MEMBRANES

Etiology

- Prelabor rupture of membranes (PROM), also known as *premature rupture of membranes*, refers to rupture of fetal membranes prior to the onset of uterine contractions.
- This can occur at term ($\geq$37 weeks of gestation) or preterm (<37 weeks of gestation, called *preterm prelabor rupture of membranes [PPROM]*)

- Risk factors include amniotic infection, shortened cervix, cigarette smoking, illicit drug use, low socioeconomic status, history of bleeding during the second and third trimesters, and history of PROM or PPROM.

Epidemiology[1]

- PPROM and preterm delivery occur in about 12% of births in the United States.
- PPROM is associated with increased risk of chorioamnionitis, umbilical cord prolapse, abruptio placentae, and complications of fetal prematurity such as respiratory distress.

Clinical Presentation

- Patients will often complain of feeling a gush of fluid from the vagina, but some women will experience a constant discharge of clear, nonodorous fluid from the vagina.

Diagnosis

- Pelvic examination must occur using a sterile speculum and sterile gloves.
- Avoid performing a digital cervical exam.
- Sometimes amniotic fluid will be visible coming out of the cervix.
- Pooling in the vaginal fornix is the pathognomonic finding in PPROM.
- Nitrazine paper will turn blue as the pH of amniotic fluid is alkalinic, but blood, semen, and some vaginal infections can turn nitrazine paper blue as well.
- Ferning is pathognomonic for amniotic fluid.
- See Box 3.3 for an overview of the diagnosis of ruptured membranes.

Management[1]

- Verify the gestational age and presentation of the fetus.
- Assessment of fetal well-being can be accomplished with an NST.
- Ultrasonic measurement of amniotic fluid is sometimes indicated.

Box 3.3 Diagnosis of Rupture of Membranes

- Amniotic fluid visualized from the cervix
- Pooling of amniotic fluid in the posterior fornix is pathognomonic
- Ferning of vaginal fluid
- Nitrazine paper turns blue (but blood, certain bacteria, and semen can cause nitrazine paper to turn blue
- Ultrasonic measurement of amniotic fluid is sometimes indicated

- If Group B *Streptococcus* status has not already been assessed, a rectovaginal swab should be performed. See "Group B Streptococcal Colonization" section in this chapter.
- In patients who are 37w0d or more, continuous monitoring of fetal heart rate and uterine contractions is advised.
- If PPROM occurs before 32w0d and there is risk for imminent delivery, magnesium sulfate should be administered as a fetal neuroprotective.
- In women with PPROM who are less than 34w0d and who are undergoing expectant management, antibiotics should be administered.
  - ○ ACOG recommends ampicillin and erythromycin intravenously, followed by oral erythromycin and amoxicillin.[1]
- In PPROM, one course of corticosteroids is recommended between 24w0d and 34w0d.[1]
  - ○ Many obstetricians will extend antenatal steroids up to 36w0d.
- In patients with PPROM at 37w0d or more, induction of labor should occur if spontaneous labor is not present.
- If there is evidence of chorioamnionitis, vaginal bleeding that could indicate an abruption, or a nonreassuring fetal heart rate pattern, consideration should be given to prompt delivery.

REFERENCE

1. American College of Obstetricians and Gynecologists. Practice bulletin no. 188. Prelabor rupture of membranes. https://www.acog.org/Clinical -Guidance-and-Publications/Practice-Bulletins/Committee-on-Practice-Bulletins -Obstetrics/Prelabor-Rupture-of-Membranes. Published January 2018.

PRETERM LABOR

Etiology

- The etiology of preterm labor is poorly understood but several theories exist. Ongoing studies may soon elucidate its underlying pathophysiology.

Epidemiology[1]

- Approximately 50% of women who deliver preterm infants experienced preterm labor symptoms prior to the delivery.

Clinical Presentation

- Patients typically present with low-back pain, mild uterine contractions, or abdominopelvic pain that patients often describe as feeling like menstrual cramps.

Diagnosis

- A diagnosis of preterm labor is made when a pregnant patient who is less than 37 weeks' gestation experiences contractions that are strong enough to cause effacement and dilation of the cervix, or dilation of the cervix to at least 2 cm with contractions.[1]
- Fetal fibronectin and cervix length measurements can be used but must be considered within the context of the clinical picture.
- Fetal fibronectin has poor positive predictive value when used alone.[1]
- A cervical length of less than 20 mm and a positive fetal fibronectin test in a patient between 22 and 34 weeks' gestation should warrant a course of corticosteroids for fetal lung maturity.[2]

Management

- The use of tocolytics, such as calcium channel blockers or beta agonists, can be considered for women less than 34 weeks' gestation who need 48 hours to complete a course of corticosteroids.[1]
- Magnesium sulfate can be considered for neuroprotection.[1]
- Women with a history of a preterm singleton delivery should be offered progesterone therapy. The current recommendation is the use of 17 alpha-hydroxyprogesterone caproate 250 mg intramuscularly (IM), weekly, starting at 16 weeks.[3]
- Women without a history of a preterm singleton delivery but who have evidence of a short cervix should be offered vaginal progesterone suppositories as soon as the cervical length has been measured and deemed short (≤20 mm by 24 weeks' gestation).[3]

> **CLINICAL PEARL:** Patients who present with symptoms suggestive of preterm labor but who have no cervical change may benefit from measurement of the cervical length to assess overall risk.

REFERENCES

1. American College of Obstetricians and Gynecologists. ACOG practice bulletin no. 171. Management of preterm labor: interim update. https://www.acog.org/Clinical -Guidance-and-Publications/Practice-Bulletins/Committee-on-Practice-Bulletins -Obstetrics/Management-of-Preterm-Labor. Published October 2016. Reaffirmed 2018.
2. Society for Maternal Fetal Medicine. When to use fetal fibronectin. https://www .smfm.org/publications/117-when-to-use-fetal-fibronectin. Reaffirmed August 2016.
3. American College of Obstetricians and Gynecologists. ACOG practice bulletin no. 130. Prediction and prevention of preterm birth. https://www.acog.org/Clinical -Guidance-and-Publications/Practice-Bulletins/Committee-on-Practice-Bulletins -Obstetrics/Prediction-and-Prevention-of-Preterm-Birth. Published October 2012. Reaffirmed 2018.

RHESUS INCOMPATIBILITY

Etiology
- ABO is the classification of human blood. Patients can be blood type A, B, O, or AB.
- The Rhesus (Rh) factor is reported as positive or negative.
- Rh antigens are proteins on the surface of red blood cells.
- Humans can have D, C, c, E, e, or G antigens. The most common is D.
- The presence of the antigen means a person is Rh (D) positive.
- Rh (D) negative people do not have the antigen.
- Rh (D) incompatibility describes the clinical scenario of a woman who is Rh (D) negative who is exposed to Rh (D) positive red blood cells and develops anti-D antibodies. This is called *alloimmunization*.
- Common causes of alloimmunization include any procedure in an Rh (D) negative woman in which fetal mixing of blood can occur, such as amniocentesis, chorionic villus sampling, and surgical management of ectopic pregnancy.
- In subsequent pregnancies, fetuses that are Rh (D) positive are at risk of developing hemolytic disease of the fetus and newborn.

Epidemiology
- The prevalence of Rh (D) negative blood varies considerably among different ethnic populations.
- Up to 35% of Basques and 15% of North American or European Caucasians are Rh (D) negative.

Clinical Presentation
- Patients are asymptomatic and screening during pregnancy identifies patients who are at risk or previously experienced alloimmunization.

Diagnosis
- All gravid women must be screened for Rh (D) negative blood and the presence of anti-Rh (D) antibodies.
- Screening is done on all women at the first prenatal visit and again at 28 weeks.
- The antibody screen is also called the *indirect Coombs test*.

Management
- If maternal alloimmunization occurs, patients should be referred to a maternal–fetal medicine specialist.
- Monitoring of these patients includes serial anti-D titers and ultrasonography of the fetal middle cerebral artery (MCA) peak systolic velocity.
- Increased MCA velocity is indicative of fetal anemia.

- Sequelae of untreated Rh incompatibility can lead to erythroblastosis fetalis.
  - Fetuses will develop ascites, heart failure, and pericardial effusion.
- Fetal hydrops is the presence of at least two of the following: a pleural effusion, pericardial effusion, ascites, increased skin and/or placental thickness, and polyhydramnios.[2]
- If in utero death does not occur, the newborn can develop kernicterus due to the inability of the liver to conjugate the high levels of resultant bilirubin.
- Fetal transfusion can be initiated when fetal hematocrit is less than 30% up until 30 to 32 weeks' gestation with plan for delivery between 32 and 34 weeks.[1]
- Prevention of alloimmunization is accomplished by giving the Rh (D)-negative gravid patient one 300-mcg dose of anti-D immunoglobulin at 28 weeks' gestation and again postpartum if the fetus is Rh (D) positive.
- In Rh (D) patients who experience a first-trimester pregnancy loss and/or uterine instrumentation prior to 12 weeks' gestation, a 50-mcg dose of anti-D immunoglobulin can be given.

> **CLINICAL PEARL:** Patients who are Rh negative who have a positive antibody screen do not need a RhoGAM injection because they have already undergone alloimmunization. However, they need to be referred to a maternal–fetal medicine specialist.

REFERENCES

1. American College of Obstetricans and Gynecologists. Practice bulletin no. 181. Prevention of Rh D alloimmunization. https://www.acog.org/Clinical-Guidance-and-Publications/Practice-Bulletins/Committee-on-Practice-Bulletins-Obstetrics/Prevention-of-Rh-D-Alloimmunization. Published August 2017.
2. Cacciatore A, Rapiti S, Carrara S, et al. Obstetric management in Rh alloimmunized pregnancy. *J Prenat Med.* 2009;3(2):25–27. https://www.prenatalmedicine.com/common/php/portiere.php?ID=d57584d14d39ce0b41b12b31c04d5eb4

SEIZURE DISORDER

Etiology

- Epilepsy is also called *epileptic seizure disorder*.
- Most cases of epilepsy are considered idiopathic, meaning no identifiable structural abnormality or other pathology can be identified.
- Other pathologies that can cause seizures include brain masses, congenital malformations, and even strokes.[1]
- Seizures that occur due to a known etiology, such as a structural issue, is considered symptomatic or secondary epilepsy[1]

- CNS infections can cause seizures.
  - ○ These are referred to as *nonepileptic seizures*.
- Other causes of symptomatic seizures include the following:
  - ○ Head trauma
  - ○ Cerebral hypoxia
  - ○ Autoimmune disorders
  - ○ Metabolic abnormalities, such as hypocalcemia, hyponatremia, and hypoglycemia
  - ○ Drug withdrawal

Epidemiology

- Over one million women of childbearing age have a seizure disorder.[2]
- Women with an epileptic seizure disorder have a 10-fold increased risk of overall mortality.[3]
- Women with an epileptic seizure disorder are at greater risk of cesarean delivery, preeclampsia, premature delivery, PPROM, and postpartum hemorrhage.[3]
- Women who take antiepileptic drugs are at risk for small-for-gestational-age fetuses, low-birth-weight infants, microcephalic infants, low Apgar scores, and the need fo neonatal intensive care.[3]
- Seizure disorders can worsen in pregnancy due to the physiological changes associated with pregnancy, which result in pharmacokinetic alterations.[3]

Clinical Presentation[1]

- Patients usually present to their obstetrician-gynecologists with a history of a seizure disorder.
- It is important to recognize status epilepticus, as prompt treatment is required.
- Status epilepticus can present as convulsive or nonconvulsive.
- Generalized convulsive status epilepticus is characterized by a tonic–clonic seizure that lasts longer than 5 to 10 minutes, or two or more seizures that occur without the patient regaining consciousness.
- Patients who present with generalized tonic–clonic seizures in the absence of a history of a seizure disorder who are in their second or third trimester and have a history of elevated BP are considered to be eclamptic.

Diagnosis

- A thorough history and physical examination should be completed.
- History must include presence or absence of prior seizures and risks for seizures.
- Risks for seizures include illicit drug use, alcohol withdrawal, prior head trauma, current CNS infections, and medications prescribed for a known seizure disorder.

- It may also be helpful to identify known triggers for seizures, including flashing lights.
- Patients who present acutely must undergo a thorough physical examination.
  - Elements of the physical exam in the acute presentation that are essential include the following:[1]
    - Inspection of the head for evidence of trauma
    - Inspection of the oral mucosa for trauma
    - Fundoscopy to assess for papilledema
    - Neck stiffness
      - Neck stiffness is associated with meningitis and subarachnoid hemorrhage.
  - Neurological exam must document the presence or absence of focal neurological deficits and hyperreflexia.
- A neurological consult is imperative in patients who present with a new-onset seizure.
- Ancillary testing of nonpregnant patients with new-onset seizures include lumbar puncture, neuroimaging, and EEG.
- Patients who present with generalized tonic–clonic seizures in the absence of a history of a seizure disorder who are in their second or third trimester and have a history of elevated BPs are considered to be eclamptic.
- The classification of epileptic seizure disorders is categorized as generalized or partial.[4]
- Generalized seizures can cause loss of consciousness and are usually followed by a postictal state.
- Examples of generalized seizures include the following:
  - Tonic
  - Tonic–clonic
  - Atonic
  - Absence
- Partial seizures include the following:
  - Simple, without loss of consciousness
  - Complex, with altered level of consciousness but no complete loss of consciousness
- Many patients will experience an aura prior to a seizure event.

Management

- Generalized seizures that last longer than 60 minutes are associated with poor outcomes, including permanent brain damage and even death.[1]
- The management of eclampsia can be found in "Eclampsia" earlier in this chapter.
- Patients of reproductive age who are not pregnant but may wish to conceive must be counseled on the risks and benefits of continuing their antiseizure medications.

- Lamotrigine, levetiracetam, and oxcarbazepine are commonly used in pregnancy.[2]
- Antiseizure medications must be monitored during pregnancy due to pharmacokinetic changes during pregnancy.[2]
- Certain antiepileptics should be avoided in pregnancy due their association with significant adverse fetal effects.[2]
  - These drugs include valproic acid, phenobarbital, carbamazepine, phenytoin, primidone, and topiramate.
- If patients present at their initial obstetric visit and are taking any of the drugs listed as being associated with adverse fetal effects, the patient should be promptly referred to maternal–fetal medicine for counseling regarding the risk of congenital anomalies.
- Patients of reproductive age and pregnant patients must be counseled to take 4 mg of folic acid each day.
- Patients should be referred to maternal–fetal medicine for a level II ultrasound at around 18 to 20 weeks.
- Seizure prophylaxis with intravenous diazepam may be considered during labor and delivery.

CLINICAL PEARL: Antiseizure medications are often used to treat other disorders besides seizures, such as neuropathy and migraines. Always review the patient's medication list to be sure not to miss a potential teratogen.

REFERENCES

1. Adamolekun B. Seizure disorders. *Merck Manual Professional Version*. Kenilworth, NJ: Merck Sharp & Dohme Corp. https://www.merckmanuals.com/professional/neurologic-disorders/seizure-disorders/seizure-disorders. Updated November 2018.
2. Patel SI, Pennell PG. Management of epilepsy during pregnancy: an update. *Ther Adv Neurol Disord*. 2016;9(2):118–129. doi:10.1177/1756285615623934
3. MacDonald S, Bateman B, McElrath T, Hernández-Díaz S. Mortality and morbidity during delivery hospitalization among pregnant women with epilepsy in the United States. *JAMA Neurol*. 2015;72:981–988. doi:10.1001/jamaneurol.2015.1017
4. Berg AT, Berkovic SF, Brodie MJ, et al. Revised terminology and concepts for organization of seizures and epilepsies: report of the ILAE (International League Against Epilepsy) commission on classification and terminology, 2005–2009. *Epilepsia*. 2010;51:676–685. doi:10.1111/j.1528-1167.2010.02522.x

SHOULDER DYSTOCIA

Etiology

- Shoulder dystocia occurs when the fetal shoulders impede passage through the maternal pelvis once the head has been delivered.
- Shoulder dystocia can occur with fetal macrosomia and precipitous delivery.
- Shoulder dystocia is associated with a greater risk of postpartum hemorrhage and a higher degree of perineal injuries.

Epidemiology

- Up to 3% of vaginal deliveries are complicated by shoulder dystocia.
- Shoulder dystocia can occur in otherwise normal pregnancies in the absence of fetal macrosomia or maternal diabetes.

Clinical Presentation

- Once the fetal head has been delivered, recurrent retraction of the head (called the *turtle sign*) may suggest shoulder dystocia but is not pathognomonic.
- Inability to deliver the fetus after various retraction methods have been used strongly suggests shoulder dystocia.

Diagnosis

- The diagnosis is made clinically by the presence of recurrent retraction of the head and an inability to deliver the fetus despite use of retraction methods.

Management

- The McRoberts maneuver should be the first maneuver attempted once shoulder dystocia is suspected.
  - The McRoberts maneuver requires two people, each flexing the patient's thighs against the abdomen.
  - If the dystocia is not relieved, downward and lateral suprapubic pressure is applied in order to displace the fetal shoulder.
- Delivery should not be rushed when dystocia is suspected. It is helpful to let the infant's head "supercrown" for a number of contractions to increase the probability that the shoulder will spontaneously maneuver past the symphysis pubis.
- Intervening too early does not allow further spontaneous descent, which increases the likelihood of the "turtle sign."
- The Wood's corkscrew maneuver[2] and delivery of the posterior arm often allow successful vaginal delivery when shoulder dystocia occurs.
  - Two fingers are placed in the vagina and onto the anterior aspect of the posterior shoulder.

○ Pressure is applied to extend the shoulder and rotate the fetus 180 degrees. After rotating 90 degrees, you may need to switch hands.
- Fetal brachial plexus injuries and clavicle fractures are common sequelae of shoulder dystocia.
- A smaller proportion of fetuses will suffer severe hypoxia or death.

REFERENCES

1. American College of Obstetricians and Gynecologists. Practice bulletin no. 178. Shoulder dystocia. https://www.acog.org/Clinical-Guidance-and-Publications/Practice-Bulletins/Committee-on-Practice-Bulletins-Obstetrics/Shoulder-Dystocia. Published May 2017. Reaffirmed 2019.
2. Busti AJ, ed. Woods corkscrew maneuver for shoulder dystocia. *Evidence-Based Medicine Consult*. EBM Consult, LLC. https://www.ebmconsult.com/articles/woods-corkscrew-maneuver. Updated September 2016.

THYROID DISEASE IN PREGNANCY

Etiology
- The thyroid gland undergoes physiologic changes during pregnancy.
- During the third trimester, thyroid volume may increase up to 30% from baseline.
- Thyroid function tests change during pregnancy.
  ○ During the first trimester, TSH levels may physiologically decrease due to stimulation of receptors from HCG.
  ○ During the first trimester, the decrease in TSH that occurs physiologically will cause an increase in thyroxine (T4).
  ○ Once the first trimester ends, TSH will return to baseline but gradually increases during the third trimester.

Epidemiology
- Hyperthyroidism complicates less than 1% of pregnancies.
- Hypothoyroidism complicates up to 10% of pregnancies.
- During the first year postpartum, 5% to 10% of women will develop a transient autoimmune thyroiditis.

Clinical Presentation
- Patients with hypothyroidism may present with classic signs and symptoms, including fatigue, muscle cramps, constipation, decreased deep tendon reflexes, weight gain, dry skin, and hair loss.
  ○ Some of these symptoms are indistinguishable from general pregnancy symptoms.

- Patients with hyperthyroidism may present with classic signs and symptoms, including tachycardia, palpitations, hypertension, nervousness/anxiety, frequent bowel movements, hyperhidrosis, heat intolerance, weight loss, and a goiter.
- Graves' disease typically manifests with exophthalmos, lid lag, and lid retraction.
  - Patients may have myxedema.
- Patients with thyroid storm will have cardiovascular, CNS, thermoregulatory, and GI dysfunction.

Diagnosis

- It is not recommended to screen pregnant women who do not have a history of thyroid disease or symptoms of hyper- or hypothyroidism.
- Initial testing for thyroid dysfunction should begin with TSH.
- If TSH levels are abnormal, subsequent measurement of T4 is advised.
- As is true in the nonpregnant patient, elevated TSH with a low free T4 is hypothyroidism.
- As is true in the nonpregnant patient, decreased TSH with an elevated free T4 is hyperthyroidism.
- Thyroid storm can be fatal so prompt treatment is advised.
  - Laboratory testing will reveal elevated T3 and T4 with low TSH.
  - Hypercalcemia can occur.
- Postpartum thyroiditis can occur up to 1 year postdelivery.
  - Patients who develop postpartum thyroiditis are at risk for developing hypothyroidism.

Management

- It is important to treat hypothyroidism and hyperthyroidism in pregnancy.
- Untreated hypothyroidism in pregnancy is associated with early pregnancy loss/spontaneous abortion, preeclampsia, preterm delivery, and abruptio placentae.
- Untreated hyperthyroidism in pregnancy is associated with fetal hydrops, intrauterine growth restriction, preterm delivery, low birth weight, and fetal thyroid dysfunction.
- Propylthiouracil (PTU) or methimazole can be used to treat hyperthyroidism in pregnancy.
  - Treatment during the first trimester is with PTU.
  - Treatment in the second and third trimesters is with methimazole.
  - PTU is associated with hepatotoxicity and methimazole has been associated with rare birth defects.
- Treatment of hypothyroidism is with levothyroxine.
  - A starting dose of 1 to 2 mcg/kg/d (100 mcg/d) is recommended.
  - Women who are s/p thyroidectomy or thyroid ablation may require increased dosing.

○ In patients with preexisting hypothyroidism, an increase of levothyroxine by 25% is recommended at the patient's first prenatal visit.
- All women should be counseled on iodine requirements during the reproductive life span.
  ○ Nonpregnant women should have a daily intake of 150 mcg of iodine.
  ○ Pregnant women should have a daily intake of 220 mcg of iodine.
  ○ Lactating women should have a daily intake of 290 mcg of iodine.

REFERENCE

1. American College of Obstetricians and Gynecologists. ACOG practice bulletin no. 148. Thyroid disease in pregnancy. https://www.acog.org/Clinical-Guidance-and-Publications/Practice-Bulletins/Committee-on-Practice-Bulletins-Obstetrics/Thyroid-Disease-in-Pregnancy. Published April 2015. Reaffirmed 2017.

VENOUS THROMBOEMBOLISM

Etiology[1,2]
- Pregnancy is a hypercoagulable state.
- Virchow's triad is present in pregnancy as evidenced by the hypercoagulable state resulting from coagulation protein changes, venous turbulence and stasis, and endothelial dysfunction.[1]
- Fibrinogen; factors VII, VIII, and X; Von Willebrand factor; and plasminogen activator inhibitors 1 and 2 are all increased during pregnancy.
- Protein C and protein S resistance develops during pregnancy.[1]
- Patients may have an underlying coagulopathy.[2]
- Thrombophilias in pregnancy can increase a patient's risk of developing a venous thromboembolic event (VTE).[2]
- Low-risk thrombophilias include factor V Leiden (heterozygote), protein C or protein S deficiency, and antiphospholipid antibody.[2]
- High-risk thrombophilias include factor V Leiden (homozygote) and antithrombin deficiency.[2]

Epidemiology[2]
- VTE occurs in almost 10% of pregnancies.
- About 80% of thromboembolic events are venous.
- VTE in pregnancy is caused by deep vein thrombosis in 75% to 80% of cases.
- Twenty percent to 25% of VTE in pregnancy is due to pulmonary embolism (PE).
- Risk of a VTE event is highest during the first week postpartum.
- Risks for VTE in pregnancy include a history of a VTE and acquired or inherited thrombophilia.
- Patients with a history of a VTE are up to four times as likely to develop another VTE in pregnancy.

Presentation

- The presentation of VTE in pregnancy is similar to that in the nonpregnant state.
- A pregnant patient who presents with unilateral lower extremity pain and swelling must be ruled out for a DVT.
- A pregnant patient who presents with an acute onset of shortness of breath must be ruled out for a PE.

Diagnosis

- Diagnosis of DVT is with compression ultrasonography of the lower extremity.
- Diagnosis of PE is with CT angiography.

Management[1,2]

- Low-molecular-weight heparin is the recommended treatment of VTE in pregnancy.
- Anti-Xa inhibitors and oral direct thrombin inhibitors have not demonstrated safety in pregnancy or breastfeeding and should not be used.
- Enoxaparin 1 mg/kg every 12 hours is the most commonly used low-molecular-weight heparin for VTE in pregnancy.
  - Enoxaparin should not be used in patients with creatine clearance less than 30 mL/min.
- Unfractionated heparin can be used if the patient is likely to have a surgical procedure because it is easily reversible with protamine.
  - Unfractionated heparin should be given in at least 10,000 units twice a day to achieve an aPTT of 1.5 to 2.5 × control.
  - Unfractionated heparin has a shorter half-life than low-molecular-weight heparin.
- In women who develop heparin-induced thrombocytopenia, fondaparinux can be used.
- The prophylaxis of patients at risk of developing a VTE includes the following:
  - A low-molecular-weight heparin, such as enoxaparin, 40 mg subcutaneously every day
  - Unfractionated heparin dosing:
    - 5,000 to 7,500 units twice daily during the first trimester
    - 7,500 to 10,000 units twice daily during the second trimester
    - 10,000 units twice daily during the third trimester, unless the aPTT is prolonged
- It is recommended that women who are undergoing a surgical procedure, discontinue anticoagulation at least 12 hours prior to surgery.
- If vaginal delivery is induced, low-molecular-weight heparin or unfractionated heparin can be discontinued 24 hours prior to the induction.
- Resumption of anticoagulation can begin no earlier than 4 to 6 hours after a vaginal delivery or 6 to 12 hours after a cesarean delivery.

- All women should have pneumatic compression devices in place before surgery and until the patient becomes ambulatory.

> **CLINICAL PEARL:** As pregnancy is a hypercoagulable state, patients who present with any signs or symptoms suggestive of a DVT or PE must be ruled out promptly. Remember that the Homan's sign has poor predictive value and should not be used to guide an evaluation.

REFERENCES

1. Springel EH. Thromboembolism in pregnancy. In: Ramus RM, ed. *Medscape.* https://emedicine.medscape.com/article/2056380-overview. Updated June 7, 2018.
2. American College of Obstetricians and Gynecologists. ACOG practice bulletin no. 196. Thromboembolism in pregnancy. https://www.acog.org/Clinical-Guidance-and-Publications/Practice-Bulletins/Committee-on-Practice-Bulletins-Obstetrics/Thromboembolism-in-Pregnancy. Published June 25, 2018.

ZIKA INFECTION IN PREGNANCY

Etiology[1,2]

- Zika is a flavivirus, similar to dengue and chikungunya.
- Zika is transmitted to humans via an infected *Aedes* mosquito.
- It can then be transferred to the fetus during pregnancy and through sexual contact.
- Transmission can also occur during laboratory preparations of samples and through blood transfusions.
- Congenital Zika syndrome describes a cluster of birth defects that can be manifested in fetuses and infants of infected mothers.
- Various abnormalities that have been documented include severe microcephaly, severe microcephaly with a partial skull collapse, calcifications in the subcortical brain region, a thin cerebral cortex, retinal changes, contractures, hypertonia, and extrapyramidal effects.
- Zika has also been linked to pregnancy loss and stillbirth.

Epidemiology[1,2]

- Zika can be found in the southeastern United States, Mexico, the Caribbean, South America, Central America, the Pacific Islands, and parts of Africa and Asia.

Clinical Presentation[2]

- Many patients will be asymptomatic; therefore it is important to screen women for possible exposure at every prenatal visit.

- Any person who traveled to or resided in a Zika endemic area and any person with an acute onset of fever, arthralgia, conjunctivitis, and rash, is considered to have possible exposure to Zika.
- Only about 20% of patients who test positive for Zika will have these symptoms.
- Although these symptoms are nonspecific, follow-up with confirmatory labs is essential (see "Diagnosis" section).
- Partners of pregnant patients should also be screened as transmission during pregnancy can occur.

Diagnosis[1]

- Every patient should be reassessed for her risk of Zika infection at each prenatal visit.
- Remember to ask about possible exposure even prior to the current pregnancy.
- Serologic testing for immunoglobulin M (IgM) and nucleic acid tests are the current testing modalities most commonly used.
- Zika testing with amniocentesis can be accomplished using nucleic acid testing.
- Serial ultrasounds in high-risk patients can also help stratify or confirm the diagnosis.
- Testing with IgM has several limitations:
  - Because Zika is a flavivirus like dengue and chikungunya, there can be cross-reactivity with IgM testing.
  - Evidence of Zika via IgM can last as long as 4 months. This makes it challenging to conclude whetherthe infection is recent.
  - IgM sensitivity and specificity become worse as prevalence decreases.
- All women who undergo Zika testing must be counseled about the limitations of current testing, including serology, nucleic acid tests, and ultrasonography.

Management[1]

- Prevention of Zika infection is of utmost importance.
- All pregnant women, women wishing to conceive, and their partners should avoid travel to Zika endemic areas.
- If travel is necessary, it is important to take steps to prevent mosquito bites, including use of diethyltoluamide (DEET), keeping exposed areas covered, avoiding the outdoors, and using permethrin on clothing.
- Other preventive measures include using condoms or abstaining if a partner travels to or lives in a Zika endemic area.
- Ultrasonography can be used to evaluate the potentially affected fetus.
- Common imaging findings in Zika include microcephaly, ventriculomegaly, and other brain anomalies.

- Ultrasonography has limited positive and negative predictive value and must be discussed with the patient at risk.
- The CDC maintains up-to-date information about Zika (www.cdc.gov/zika).

REFERENCES

1. American College of Obstetricians and Gynecologists. Practice advisory: interim guidance for care of obstetric patients during a Zika virus outbreak. Washington, DC: American College of Obstetricians and Gynecologists. https://www.acog.org/Clinical-Guidance-and-Publications/Practice-Advisories/Practice-Advisory-Interim-Guidance-for-Care-of-Obstetric-Patients-During-a-Zika-Virus-Outbreak#Figure%201%20sep%202017. Updated September 13, 2017.
2. Centers for Disease Control and Prevention. Zika virus. https://www.cdc.gov/zika

4

Diagnostic Testing for OB/GYN Conditions

Introduction

While not meant to be exhaustive, this chapter presents some of the most common laboratory and imaging testing you may encounter. Always remember to correlate laboratory and imaging findings with your history and physical examination.

COMMON LABORATORY TESTS

ABO AND RHESUS FACTOR

TABLE 4.1 ABO and Rhesus Factor

Name	Normal Reference Range	Indication	Interpretation
ABO	A, B, O, or AB	Pregnancy Hemorrhage	N/A
Rh	Negative or positive	Pregnancy Hemorrhage	Positive: no need for Rho(D) immunoglobulin Negative: will need antibody screen and, if negative, administer Rho(D) immunoglobulin at 28 weeks and delivery (if fetus is Rh positive)

Rh, Rhesus factor.

ANTIBODY SCREEN

TABLE 4.2 Antibody Screen (Indirect Coombs Test)

Name	Normal Reference Range	Indication	Interpretation
Antibody screen	Negative, no antibody detected	Pregnancy	If positive, could indicate potential for the development of fetal hydrops. Further testing to identify the antibody is completed. Antibodies to Duffy, Kell, Kidd, MNS, and P are generally considered to be clinically significant. IgG antibodies are considered more significant than IgM antibodies. Refer to maternal–fetal medicine specialist. Once levels reach a critical threshold (usually ≥1:32), Doppler velocimetry is performed on the fetal middle cerebral artery. High velocity correlates with severe fetal anemia.

IgG, immunoglobulin G; IgM, immunoglobulin M.

CLINICAL PEARL: The antibody screen is done at the initial prenatal visit and again between 26 to 28 weeks.

ANTI-MÜLLERIAN HORMONE

TABLE 4.3 Common Laboratory Test: Anti-Müllerial Hormone

Name	Normal Reference Range	Indication	Interpretation
AMH	<24 months: <4.7 ng/mL 24 months–12 years: <8.8 ng/mL 13–45 years: 0.9 to 9.5 ng/mL >45 years: <1.0 ng/mL	Assessment of menopausal status and ovarian function	Low AMH is associated with reproductive decline. Elevated AMH generally means a better response to ovarian stimulation. Women with PCOS may have an elevated AMH (sometimes 2–5 times the reference range).

AMH, anti-Müllerian hormone; PCOS, polycystic ovarian syndrome.

CLINICAL PEARL: Before sending a patient to a reproductive endocrinologist for an infertility workup, make sure you have ordered an anti-Müllerian hormone (AMH) along with the rest of the appropriate work-up for infertility, including a semen analysis of the partner.

BETA HUMAN CHORIONIC GONADOTROPIN (β-HCG)

Serum human chorionic gonadotropin (HCG) can be ordered as a quantitative or qualitative test (Table 4.4). In OB/GYN, it is most useful to always order quantitative levels, particularly because measuring the rise or fall of HCG with serial blood tests helps to manage patients who are being evaluated and treated for an ectopic pregnancy, gestational trophoblastic disease (GTD), germ cell tumors of the ovary, or first-trimester bleeding. It is important to remember that correlating HCG with gestational age has limitations and must be used with ultrasound (see Table 4.5).

TABLE 4.4 Common Laboratory Test: Beta-HCG

Name	Normal Reference Range	Indication	Interpretation
Beta-HCG	<5 mIU/mL	To rule out pregnancy, follow-up in threatened abortions and ectopic pregnancies during medical management. Also used to correlate with ultrasound findings in early pregnancy (see Table 4.5).	During early pregnancy, HCG levels should double about every 48–72 hours. HCG levels fall after about 20 weeks' gestation. HCG has a half-life of 24–36 hours, so after an elective pregnancy termination, spontaneous abortion, or delivery, HCG levels will fall accordingly. If retained products of conception are present, the decline may be absent or much slower. Patients with GTD will have significantly elevated HCG. Down syndrome pregnancies will also have a significantly elevated HCG.

Beta-HCG, beta human chorionic gonadotropin; GTD, gestational trophoblastic disease.

TABLE 4.5 Correlation of Beta-HCG and Gestational Weeks

Gestational Age	Expected HCG Values (mIU/mL)
<1 week	5–50
1–2 weeks	50–500
2–3 weeks	100–5,000
3–4 weeks	500–10,000
4–5 weeks	1,000–50,000
5–6 weeks	10,000–100,000
6–8 weeks	15,000–200,000
2–3 months	10,000–100,000

Beta-HCG, beta human chorionic gonadotropin; LMP, last menstrual period.

Source: Quest Diagnostics. Hcg with gestational table. https://testdirectory.questdiagnostics.com/test/test-detail/19485/hcg-with-gestational-table?cc=MASTER

CLINICAL PEARL: Always make sure to order a quantitative HCG as a qualitative (positive or negative) test cannot be tracked over time.

CYSTIC FIBROSIS (CF) SCREEN

All pregnant women should be offered cystic fibrosis (CF) screening (Table 4.6). If CF testing indicates the patient is a carrier, the father of the baby should get tested. Two CF gene mutations, called *cystic fibrosis transmembrane conductance regulator gene mutation (CFTR)*, one from each parent, is necessary for the infant to inherit the disease. In the first pregnancy in which both parents carry the mutation, these is a 25% risk the infant will have CF, but a 50% chance the infant will become a carrier and not have active disease. The CF mutation is more prevalent among European Caucasians, and least common among Asians.[1]

TABLE 4.6 Common Laboratory Test: CF Screening

Name	Normal Reference Range	Indication	Interpretation
CF screen	CF carrier negative	To rule out CF carrier status	The most common mutation is F508del, or delta F508; current CF testing is 99% sensitive in diagnosing the presence of a mutation.

CF, cystic fibrosis.

Follicle-Stimulating Hormone (FSH)

Table 4.7 Common Laboratory Test: FSH

Name	Normal Reference Range	Indication	Interpretation
FSH	>10 years–≤15 years: 0.9–8.9 IU/L >15 years–≤18 years: 0.7–9.6 IU/L Premenopausal Follicular: 2.9–14.6 IU/L Midcycle: 4.7–23.2 IU/L Luteal: 1.4–8.9 IU/L Postmenopausal: 16.0–157.0 IU/L	To help predict ovulation when evaluating patients with infertility, and in the workup of patients with suspected hypogonadism and pituitary disorders	Elevated FSH is associated with premature ovarian failure and menopause but fluctuates throughout the menstrual cycle. A day 3 FSH is measured in women who are undergoing evaluation for fertility disorders. Decreased FSH or normal FSH can be found in PCOS. Postmenopausal women will have elevated FSH.

FSH, follicle-stimulating hormone; PCOS, polycystic ovarian syndrome.
Source: Mayo Clinic Laboratories. Follicle-stimulating hormone, serum. https://www.mayocliniclabs.com/test-catalog/Clinical+and+Interpretive/602753

Clinical Pearl: FSH should not be used as a diagnostic biomarker in perimenopause due to its fluctuations during the menstrual cycle and during perimenopause itself.

Hepatitis B Surface Antigen (HBsAg)

Table 4.8 Common Laboratory Test: HBsAg

Name	Normal Reference Range	Indication	Interpretation
HBsAg	Negative	Pregnancy	HBsAg appears between 6 and 16 weeks following hepatitis B exposure. Persistence of HBsAg for longer than 6 months can indicate chronic HBV infection or a chronic carrier state. Patients with a positive HBsAg should have a quantitative HBV DNA, HBeAg, and ALT at baseline and again at 28 weeks. Household members and sexual contacts need to be screened as well.

(continued)

TABLE 4.8 Common Laboratory Test: HBsAg (*continued*)

Name	Normal Reference Range	Indication	Interpretation
			Referral to GI or a hepatologist is recommended if the viral load is greater than 20,000 IU/mL, the ALT is >19 IU/mL, or HBeAg is positive.
			If the patient's viral load is greater than >1 million copies (200,000 IU/mL), patients should be considered for antiviral therapy at 32 weeks' gestation.
			All infants require HBIg within 12 hours of birth and the HBV vaccination series.

ALT, alanine aminotransferase; GI, gastrointestinal; HBeAg, hepatitis B e-antigen; HBIg, hepatitis B immune globulin; HBsAg, hepatitis B surface antigen; HBV, hepatitis B virus.
Source: American College of Obstetricians and Gynecologists. Practice bulletin no. 86. Viral hepatitis in pregnancy. https://www.acog.org/Clinical-Guidance-and-Publications/Practice-Bulletins/Committee-on-Practice-Bulletins-Obstetrics/Viral-Hepatitis-in-Pregnancy. Published October 2007. Reaffirmed 2018.

LUTEINIZING HORMONE (LH)

During a normal menstrual cycle, women will experience a midcycle luteinizing hormone (LH) surge that triggers ovulation (Table 4.9). This surge also signals the follicle to become a corpus luteum that produces progesterone. Progesterone helps create a hospitable endometrial environment for possible implantation of an early pregnancy. During the first few weeks of pregnancy, HCG and LH work to maintain corpus luteal progesterone secretion until the placenta begins its own progesterone production. In nonpregnancy, LH helps ovarian thecal cells produce estradiol and androgens.

TABLE 4.9 Common Laboratory Test: LH

Name	Normal Reference Range	Indication	Interpretation
LH	>6–≤11 years: ≤3.1 IU/L >11–≤14 years: ≤11.9 IU/L >14–≤18 years: 0.5–41.7 IU/L Premenopausal Follicular: 1.9–14.6 IU/L Midcycle: 12.2–118.0 IU/L Luteal: 0.7–12.9 IU/L Postmenopausal: 5.3–65.4 IU/L	Evaluation of ovulation	LH can be elevated in menopause, PCOS, and gonadic failure. LH can be decreased in hypothalamic and pituitary failure.

LH, luteinizing hormone; PCOS, polycystic ovarian syndrome.
Source: Mayo Foundation for Medical Education and Research. Luteinizing hormone. https://www.mayocliniclabs.com/test-catalog/Overview/602752

PROGESTERONE

Progesterone is secreted by the corpus luteum, the adrenal glands, and the placenta during pregnancy. Progesterone acts on the endometrium and uterus, but also the brain and the breasts. When adequate endogenous estrogen is present, progesterone will transform the endometrium from a proliferative stage to a secretory stage, allowing increased receptivity for embryonic implantation. When implantation occurs, the corpus luteum secretes progesterone to help maintain the pregnancy until the end of the first trimester when the placental progesterone dominates. If implantation does not occur, corpus luteum degradation occurs and progesterone levels fall. For more information on progesterone laboratory testing, see Table 4.10.

TABLE 4.10 Common Laboratory Test: Progesterone

Name	Normal Reference Range	Indication	Interpretation
Progesterone	≥18 years (central 90th % of healthy population) Follicular phase: ≤0.89 ng/mL Ovulation: ≤12 ng/mL Luteal phase: 1.8–24 ng/mL Postmenopausal: ≤0.20 ng/mL Pregnancy First trimester: 11–44 ng/mL Second trimester: 25–83 ng/mL Third trimester: 58–214 ng/mL	Early pregnancy	Helpful in determining whether ovulation has occurred, in the workup and management of patients undergoing infertility protocols, to evaluate the overall health of an early pregnancy, and in the follow-up of patients at risk for preterm labor who are receiving exogenous progesterone.

Source: Mayo Foundation for Medical Education and Research. Serum progesterone. https://www.mayocliniclabs.com/test-catalog/Clinical+and+Interpretive/8141

> **CLINICAL PEARL:** Serum progesterone levels are helpful when working up a patient with a possible early pregnancy loss. Serum progesterone levels less than 6.2 ng/mL have been strongly correlated with early pregnancy loss.

RAPID PLASMA REAGIN/FLUORESCENT TREPONEMAL ANTIBODY ABSORPTION

Pregnant patients who are positive for syphilis must be treated with penicillin G 2.4 million units every week for 3 weeks. If the patient has a suspected penicillin allergy, the patient can be referred to an allergist for testing and desensitization. See Table 4.11 for more information on rapid plasma reagin/fluorescent treponemal antibody absorption (RPR/FTA-ABS) testing.

> **CLINICAL PEARL:** In patients with a positive RPR, make sure to review their past medical history for any underlying diseases.

TABLE 4.11 Common Laboratory Test: RPR/FTA-ABS

Name	Normal Reference Range	Indication	Interpretation
RPR/ FTA-ABS	Nonreactive	Pregnancy, screening in at-risk patients for syphilis	Positive results are reported as a titer.
			False positives can occur in many other conditions, including mononucleosis, malaria, systemic lupus erythematosus, viral pneumonia, and other treponemal diseases, such as yaws.
			Sequential testing that shows an increase in titers, generally considered a four-fold increase from the initial test, reflects active infection.
			The FTA-ABS test is an indirect fluorescent antibody lab technique, which is used as a confirmatory test for syphilis if the RPR or VDRL is positive.
			A nonreactive FTA-ABS result means the patient does not have syphilis.

RPR/FTA-ABS, rapid plasma reagin/fluorescent treponemal antibody absorption; VDRL, Venereal Disease Research Laboratory.

RUBELLA ANTIBODY, RUBELLA IMMUNOGLOBULIN G

Rubella is also known as *German measles*. It is a member of the togavirus family and is transmitted via respiratory droplets. Rubella causes a maculopapular rash that typically starts on the face, spreads to the trunk and extremities, and is accompanied by fever and lymphadenopathy. Although infection with rubella is generally self-limited and mild, it is associated with significant adverse fetal events if a nonimmune pregnant patient is exposed within the first 4 months of gestation. The greatest risk to a pregnancy occurs if a pregnant woman is exposed during the first 12 weeks of gestation. Fetal hearing loss is the most common sequelae, followed by cataracts, congenital heart defects, and developmental delay. For information on testing for rubella, see Table 4.12.

TABLE 4.12 Common Laboratory Test: Rubella

Name	Normal Reference Range	Indication	Interpretation
Rubella IgG	≥1.0 AI	Pregnancy	A patient who has immunity will have an AI value of 1.0 or higher.
			Pregnant patients who are nonimmune must not receive the MMR vaccine because it is a live virus.
			Nonimmune pregnant patients should be advised to avoid any person with a rash until after 20 weeks' gestation.

AI, antibody index; IgG, immunoglobulin G; MMR, measles, mumps, and rubella.

> **Clinical Pearl:** Patients who are rubella nonimmune must receive adequate patient education regarding the importance of postpartum vaccination and avoiding anyone with a rash prior to 20 weeks' gestation. Documentation of the patient education provided must be entered into the medical record.

Sex Hormone Binding Globulin

Sex hormone binding globulin (SHBG) can be used to support a diagnosis of polycystic ovarian syndrome. Other uses for SHBG can be found in Table 4.13.

Table 4.13 Common Laboratory Test: SHBG

Name	Normal Reference Range	Indication	Interpretation
SHBG	18–144 nmol/L	Used to diagnose and manage women with suspected or confirmed PCOS. It can also be used to diagnose and manage women with anorexia nervosa and thyrotoxicosis.	Low SHBG is a hallmark of PCOS and insulin resistance, even in the nonobese woman. Exogenous androgen or progestins can cause a decreased SHBG. Patients with anorexia nervosa and thyrotoxicosis will have elevated SHBG.

PCOS, polycystic ovarian syndrome; SHBG, sex hormone binding globulin.

Reference

1. Cystic Fibrosis Foundation. Carrier testing for cystic fibrosis. https://www.cff.org/What-is-CF/Testing/Carrier-Testing-for-Cystic-Fibrosis. Accessed on May 11, 2018.

Diagnostic Evaluation

Amniocentesis

Amniocentesis is an invasive procedure that is usually performed between 15 and 20 weeks' gestation. It is performed by a maternal–fetal specialist. It is a sterile procedure, performed under ultrasound guidance, in which a 22-gauge spinal needle is inserted into a deep pocket of amniotic fluid, avoiding the placenta, fetal parts, and umbilical cord. Twenty to 30 mL of fluid is withdrawn and sent to a lab for genetic testing. Risks of the procedure include pregnancy loss, albeit rare, small amniotic fluid leakage, and light vaginal bleeding. If a patient is Rh negative, she will need an injection of Rh(D) immune globulin.[1]

- Indication: Some of the indications for amniocentesis include advanced maternal age, a previous abnormal screening test for aneuploidy, measurement of fetal lung maturity, and structural anomalies detected on prior ultrasound examination.
  - Pertinent findings: N/A

AMNIOTIC FLUID INDEX (AFI)

- Indication: A measurement of amniotic fluid in the deepest vertical pocket, it is used as an assessment for oligo- or polyhydramnios. Can also be measured by the four-quadrant method.[1]
  - Pertinent findings if using a single deepest pocket measurement: An AFI of less than 2 cm indicates oligohydramnios, and an AFI of more than 8 cm indicates polyhydramnios.
  - Pertinent findings if using the four-quadrant method is an AFI greater than the 95th percentile for gestational age.
  - ACOG recommends using the single deepest pocket to diagnose oligohydramnios.

BIOPHYSICAL PROFILE (BPP)

The BPP uses external fetal monitoring and ultrasound to assess fetal health. The BPP includes five components, each given a maximum score of 2 points (Table 4.14).[1]

- Indications: To assess fetal well-being, particularly in the presence of a non-reassuring NST
  - Pertinent Findings: The management of a BPP that falls below eight of 10 depends on the amniotic fluid index (AFI) and the gestational age.
    - The modified BPP consists of the NST and an amniotic fluid volume assessment.
    - The modified BPP is considered *normal* if the NST is reactive and the deepest vertical pocket of amniotic fluid is greater than 2 cm.
    - The modified BPP is considered *abnormal* if either the NST is non-reactive or the deepest vertical pocket of amniotic fluid is less than or equal to 2 cm.

CHORIONIC VILLUS SAMPLING (CVS)

Chorionic villus sampling (CVS) is performed between 10 and 13 weeks' gestation. There are two techniques used to obtain chorionic villi cells. The first involves inserting a special catheter through the cervix under ultrasound guidance, and the second involves inserting a small needle through the abdomen, also under ultrasound guidance. The benefit of CVS is that it can be done earlier in a pregnancy than amniocentesis and requires less time to process results.

TABLE 4.14 BPP for Assessing Fetal Health

Category	Score: Normal (2 pts)	Score: Abnormal (0 pts)
Fetal breathing	One or more episodes of fetal breathing lasting at least 30 seconds in 30 minutes	No episodes of fetal breathing movements lasting at least 30 seconds during a 30-minute period of observation
Fetal movement	Three or more discrete body/limb movements in 30 minutes	Less than three body/limb movements in 30 minutes
Fetal tone	One or more episodes of active extension/flexion of fetal extremity OR opening and closing the hand in 30 minutes	Slow extension with no return/slow return to flexion of a fetal extremity, or no fetal movement
AFI	More than 2 cm at the deepest vertical pocket	Less than 2 cm at the deepest vertical pocket
NST	Reactive	Nonreactive

AFI, amniotic fluid index; BPP, biophysical profile; NST, nonstress test.

Although there are reports in the literature regarding limb defects after CVS, it appears that the risk is extremely low if CVS is performed after 10 weeks' gestation. However, pregnancy loss is still considered a risk in CVS sampling. The other risk of CVS is vaginal bleeding that resolves without any intervention.[1]

- Indication: Indications for CVS include advanced maternal age and abnormal first-trimester aneuploidy screening.
  - ○ Pertinent findings: Fetal aneuploidy, karyotype

> **CLINICAL PEARL:** It is important to identify candidates for CVS early in the first trimester as the window for performing the test is narrow (between 10 and 13 weeks).

CONTRACTION STRESS TEST (CST)

- Indication: A contraction stress test (CST) is usually performed to assess a nonlaboring patient to assure the provider that the fetus is being well oxygenated. It is rarely used anymore due to risks and contraindications.[1]
  - ○ Pertinent findings: If a patient is not experiencing spontaneous contractions, intravenous oxytocin or rigorous nipple discharge can be employed. CSTs are reported as either negative, positive, equivocal, or unsatisfactory.

Doppler Velocimetry

- Indication: Umbilical artery doppler velocimetry is an ultrasound maneuver used to evaluate vascular resistance in IUGR pregnancies and other fetal anomalies, such as Rh incompatibility.[1]
  - Pertinent findings: A normal fetus displays high-velocity diastolic flow, but in IUGR, the flow will be decreased, reversed, or absent. Reversed or absent flow is associated with severe IUGR and perinatal morbidity and mortality.

Evaluations of Fetal Health

Most prenatal evaluations of fetal health begin at 32 to 34 weeks. Some of the most common indications for prenatal evaluations include the following:[1]

- Advanced maternal age
- Diabetes
- Hypertensive disorders, including gestational hypertension (HTN), chronic HTN, and preeclampsia
- Autoimmune disorders
- Poorly controlled hyperthyroidism
- Hemoglobinopathy
- Chronic renal or hepatic disease
- Cyanotic heart disease
- Fetal growth restriction
- Decreased fetal movement
- Oligohydramnios
- Postterm pregnancy (≥42 weeks) or late-term pregnancy (between 41w0d and 41w6d)
- Rh incompatibility (isoimmunization)
- Multiple gestation
- Prior poor fetal outcome

Level II Ultrasound

- Indication: A level II ultrasound is a more detailed sonographic evaluation of the fetus or fetuses. It is indicated for a variety of reasons, including a detected or suspected anomaly during an initial (level I) ultrasound, abnormal fetal aneuploidy screening, type 1 diabetes in the mother, multiple gestation, exposure to illicit drugs and/or known teratogens during the first trimester, and a history of a fetal demise. It is typically performed at 20 weeks' gestation.
  - Pertinent Findings: See the section "Ultrasound in Pregnancy."

Nonstress Test (Also Known as *Cardiotocography* and *Antenatal Fetal Surveillance*)

This test is done in the outpatient setting, or in a separate nonstress test (NST) room on the labor and delivery floor. The patient is placed in the semi-Fowler position (seated, head elevated 30 degrees). NSTs can be used after 28 weeks' gestation when the fetus' central nervous system is mature enough to respond to sympathetic and parasympathetic changes. Two belts are placed around the gravid mother's uterus. One documents fetal heart rate, and the other documents the presence of uterine contractions. The mother holds a device that she clicks whenever she feels the baby move. A notch is recorded on the paper strip, and the evaluator can assess the fetal heart rate's reaction to its own movement or a uterine contraction.[1]

- Indication: For most indications, NST and biophysical profiles begin at 32 weeks. In some patients with severe anomalies, testing could be initiated at 26 weeks. There is little consensus regarding how often to perform NSTs and biophysical profiles (BPPs), but they are usually done either every week or twice a week. Common indications for an NST include decreased fetal movement as reported by the mother and the presence of comorbid medical problems, such as hypertension, preeclampsia, diabetes, and autoimmune disorders. Some providers will have women who are considered to be at advanced maternal age (>35 years) undergo routine NSTs starting at 32 weeks' gestation.
  - Pertinent findings:[1,2]
    - A *reactive NST* occurs when the fetal heart rate accelerates at least twice in 20 minutes, but sometimes it is appropriate to monitor for 40 minutes, depending on the sleep–wake cycle of the fetus. An acceleration is an increase in fetal heart greater than or equal to 15 beats above baseline lasting for ≥15 seconds.
    - A *nonreactive NST* occurs when the fetal heart rate does not accelerate after 40 minutes. Sometimes vibroacoustic stimulation can help elicit accelerations. A vibroacoustic device is placed on the gravid abdomen and stimulation is applied for 2 seconds. If there is still no acceleration, a repeat stimulation for 3 seconds can be performed. If the NST remains nonreactive, a biophysical profile (see text that follows) is performed.

PERIPARTUM CONTINUOUS EXTERNAL FETAL MONITORING

Continuous external fetal monitoring during labor is done at most hospitals throughout the United States and can provide valuable information about the overall health of the fetus. The exact intervention varies and depends on the condition of the mother and the fetus; as such, the entire clinical picture must be assessed.[2]

- Indication: To continuously assess the overall health of the fetus
  - Pertinent findings:
    - Fetal tachycardia: Fetal heart rate greater than 160 bpm for 10 minutes or more
      - Common causes: Maternal fever, certain drugs, infection, and dehydration

- Fetal bradycardia: Fetal heart rate less than 100 bpm for 10 minutes or more
  - Common causes: Hypoxia from cord prolapse or compression, uterine hyperstimulation, placental abruption, and uterine rupture
  - Of note, fetal bradycardia is the most common finding during a trial of labor after cesarean (TOLAC) when uterine rupture occurs
- Variability: Changes in the fetal heart rate from baseline
  - *Minimal variability*: This refers to a change less than or equal to 5 bpm or absent change from baseline; can indicate fetal hypoxia and/or metabolic acidosis.
  - *Moderate variability*: Refers to changes of 6 to 25 bpm from baseline. This is a reassuring finding.
  - *Marked variability*: Refers to changes of more than 25 bpm from baseline. The entire clinical picture must be assessed. Sometimes changing the maternal position corrects the marked variability.
- Acceleration: Refers to an increase in fetal heart of 15 beats or more above baseline lasting for 15 seconds or longer.
  - Common causes: Acceleration is a normal and reassuring finding. Lack of accelerations could be due to fetal sleep cycle or if the mother has a beta-blocker, magnesium sulfate, or opioid in her system.
- Deceleration: This refers to a transient decrease in the fetal heart rate (Figures 4.1 and 4.2).

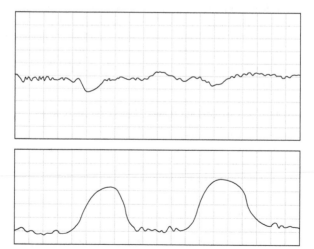

Figure 4.1 Fetal heart rate variability (top graph). Uterine contractions (bottom graph).

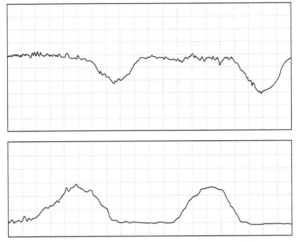

Figure 4.2   Fetal heart rate decelerations (top graph). Uterine contractions (bottom graph). Notice how the heart rate drops after the contractions. These are called late decelerations.

- Decelerations that last for 1 minute or longer are associated with poor fetal outcomes, including fetal demise and risk for cesarean delivery.
  - *Early deceleration*: This is a decrease in fetal heart rate no more than 15 bpm below the baseline, lasting longer than 15 seconds and less than 2 minutes; occurs with contractions; nadir of deceleration corresponds with peak of uterine contraction. Is usually due to head compression during labor and is a reassuring finding.
  - *Late deceleration*: This refers to a decrease of no more than 15 bpm below the baseline, lasting longer than 15 seconds and less than 2 minutes; begins after the uterine contraction has begun and nadir occurs after the contraction peaks; heart rate does not return to baseline. This finding can be due to uteroplacental insufficiency, usually due to fetal hypoxia, but can occur in uterine hyperstimulation.
  - *Variable deceleration*: This refers to a fetal heart rate decrease of more than 15 bpm below the baseline, lasts longer than 15 seconds but less than 2 minutes; usually due to umbilical cord compression. Variable decelerations that are less than 30 seconds and nonrepetitive are not associated with poor fetal outcomes. Variable decelerations that occur at least three times in 20 minutes are associated with risk of cesarean delivery. If variable decelerations are consistently occurring and do not respond to basic interventions, such as repositioning

of the mother and a vaginal exam to ensure gross cord pathology is not present, there is a risk of fetal hypoxia.

○ *Prolonged decelerations*: This refers to a fetal heart rate decrease of 15 bpm or more below baseline that lasts 2 minutes or longer. Can be due to uteroplacental insufficiency and/or cord compression. Check for cord prolapse and reposition mother. Adequate hydration, oxygenation, and decreased uterine stimulation of the mother is essential.

> **CLINICAL PEARL:** One of the best ways to learn how to interpret cardiotocographic tracings is by spending a shift with an experienced labor and delivery nurse or certified nurse midwife. It can be difficult to learn how to read NSTs and continuous tracings from a textbook.

ULTRASOUND IN PREGNANCY

- Indication: Common reasons for a first-trimester ultrasound include, but are not limited to, estimating gestational age, assessing for viability of pregnancy, screening for fetal anomalies, and to rule out pathology such as an ectopic pregnancy or molar pregnancy. First-trimester ultrasounds will also include an evaluation of the maternal uterus, cervix, and adnexa. Common indications for a second-trimester ultrasound include, but are not limited to, evaluating the growth of the fetus, screening for fetal anomalies, evaluating fetal anatomy, evaluating the placenta, measuring cervical length, and evaluating for size and date discrepancies.
  ○ Pertinent findings:
    - CRL: Crown–rump length, a first-trimester measurement, is most accurate for determining gestational age
    - BPD: Biparietal diameter
    - AC: Abdominal circumference
    - FL: Femur (femoral diaphysis) length, can be used for dating a pregnancy after 14 weeks
    - HC: Head circumference
    - AFI: Amniotic fluid index
    - EFW: Estimated fetal weight, based on a calculation with the BPD, HC, FL, and AC. EFW can have a margin of error up to 20%
    - Common sonographic findings in trisomy 21: Increased nuchal thickness, cardiac anomalies such as tetralogy of Fallot and septal defects, and duodenal atresia

> **CLINICAL PEARL:** Many patients request to know the gender of their fetus. An ultrasound can be done at 16 weeks in order to check the gender.

REFERENCES

1. American College of Obstetricians and Gynecologists. Practice bulletin no. 145. Antepartum fetal surveillance. https://www.acog.org/Clinical%20Guidance%20 and%20Publications/Practice%20Bulletins/Committee%20on%20Practice%20 Bulletins%20Obstetrics/Antepartum%20Fetal%20Surveillance.aspx. Published July 2014. Reaffirmed 2019.
2. Menihan CA, Kopel E. *Electronic Fetal Monitoring: Concepts and Applications.* 2nd ed. Philadelphia, PA: Lippincott Williams and Wilkins; 2008.

FETAL ANEUPLOIDY SCREENING

See Table 4.15 for a review of aneuploidy screening.

TABLE 4.15 Screening for Fetal Aneuploidy

	First-Trimester Screen	Second Trimester—Triple Screen	Second Trimester—Quad Screen
Dates	10–13 weeks	15–22 weeks	15–22 weeks (16–18 weeks preferred)
Serum	HCG, PAPP-A	uE3, msAFP, HCG	uE3, msAFP, HCG, inhibin A
Imaging	Nuchal translucency	Full fetal survey (18–22 weeks)	Full fetal survey (18–22 weeks)

HCG, human chorionic gonadotropin; msAFP, maternal serum alpha-fetoprotein; PAPP-A, pregnancy-associated plasma protein A; uE3, unconjugated estriol.

CELL-FREE DNA

- Indication: Cell-free DNA testing can be used to evaluate a pregnant patient for fetal aneuploidy but should never be used alone. It can also be used for fetal gender determination, the Rh status of the fetus, and to detect some autosomal dominant genetic diseases. Screening can begin at 10 weeks' gestation and has high sensitivity and specificity for the detection of trisomy 21 (Down syndrome) and trisomy 18. Cell-free DNA testing does not help to diagnose neural tube defects or other abnormalities.[1]
- Interpretation/pertinent findings: Women with indeterminate, uninterpretable, or unreported results should undergo genetic counseling and further diagnostic testing due to an increased risk of fetal aneuploidy. A negative cell-free DNA test does not rule out the presence of all fetal aneuploidies. As such, American College of Obstetricians and Gynecologists (ACOG) does not recommend cell-free DNA testing as the first choice for prenatal screening for fetal aneuploidy.

INHIBIN A

- Indication: Inhibin A is another biomarker used in second-trimester (14–16 weeks' gestation) screening for fetal aneuploidy.[2]
- Interpretation/pertinent findings: When inhibin A is combined with HCG, msAFP, and unconjugated estriol (uE3), it is called *quad testing*. Elevated levels are associated with trisomy 21.

MATERNAL SERUM ALPHA-FETOPROTEIN (MSAFP)

- Indication: Used to screen a pregnant patient for fetal aneuploidy.[2]
- Interpretation/pertinent findings: The fetal liver produces alpha-fetoprotein (AFP), and levels rise during the second trimester, particularly at 16 weeks. Results are expressed as multiples of the median (MoMs) and are dependent on each gestational week. MoMs that are 2.5 or greater are considered elevated. It is imperative that the patient's estimated due date, and hence her gestational age, are accurate, as well as her age, weight, race, and whether the patient is diabetic.
  - ○ Maternal serum alpha-fetoprotein (msAFP) can be elevated in the presence of open neural tube defects, such as anencephaly, spina bifida, and an abdominal wall defect. If the fetus has Down syndrome, the msAFP is usually lower by about 25%.

NUCHAL TRANSLUCENCY

- Indication: Nuchal translucency (NT) measurement assesses the fluid-filled space on the dorsal aspect of the neck of the fetus between 10w3d and 13w6d.[2]
- Interpretation/pertinent findings: An increased NT is strongly associated with trisomy 21 and other aneuploidies. NT is combined with serum HCG and pregnancy-associated plasma protein A (PAPP-A) in the first trimester. NT should only be performed by a certified ultrasonographer or OB/GYN.

PREGNANCY-ASSOCIATED PLASMA PROTEIN A (PAPP-A)

- Indication: It is combined with HCG and NT in the first-trimester screen (between 10 and 13 weeks' gestation).[2]
- Interpretation/pertinent findings: There have been reports in the literature that there is an association between low first-trimester PAPP-A levels and adverse outcomes, such as intrauterine growth restriction (IUGR), preterm delivery, and preeclampsia, but ACOG does not currently endorse its use as a predictive tool for those conditions. High levels of PAPP-A are currently not associated with any adverse pregnancy outcomes. A low level of PAPP-A is associated with trisomy 21.

UNCONJUGATED ESTRIOL (uE3)

- Indication: UE3 is used in conjunction with AFP, HCG, and inhibin A during the second trimester for aneuploidy screening.[2]
- Interpretation/pertinent findings: Low uE3 is associated with trisomy 21 and 18, anencephaly, Smith-Lemli-Opitz syndrome, fetal adrenal insufficiency, and is also associated with pregnancy loss. High levels may be seen in congenital adrenal hyperplasia and is also associated with onset of labor in 4 weeks. As such, it is being studied for its utility as a biomarker for preterm labor risk assessment.
- Combined first- and second-trimester screening protocols:
  - ○ *Integrated*: First-trimester screen (NT, PAPP-A) between 10 and 13w6d, then quad screen (HCG, msAFP, uE3, inhibin A) between 15 and 22 weeks. Highest trisomy 21 detection rate.
  - ○ *Serum integrated*: PAPP-A but no NT measurement between 10 and 13w6d, followed by quad screen (HCG, msAFP, uE3, inhibin A) between 15 and 22 weeks.
  - ○ *Sequential stepwise*: First-trimester screen (NT, HCG, PAPP-A) between 10 and 13w6d, then quad screen (HCG, msAFP, uE3, inhibin A) between 15 and 22 weeks.
- Increased NT, low PAPP-A, elevated inhibin A, low uE3, and low msAFP are associated with trisomy 21.
- Very low HCG, low PAPP-A, and increased NT are associated with trisomy 18.

CLINICAL PEARLS:
- Trisomy 21 is the most common autosomal trisomy.
- Klinefelter syndrome (47, XXY) is the most common sex chromosome aneuploidy.
- Turner syndrome (45, X) is the only viable monosomy.

REFERENCES

1. American College of Obstetricians and Gynecologists. Committee opinion no. 640. Cell-free DNA screening for fetal aneuploidy. https://www.acog.org/Clinical -Guidance-and-Publications/Committee-Opinions/Committee-on-Genetics/Cell -free-DNA-Screening-for-Fetal-Aneuploidy. Published September 2015.
2. American College of Obstetricians and Gynecologists. Practice bulletin no. 163. Screening for fetal aneuploidy. https://www.acog.org/Clinical%20Guidance%20and %20Publications/Practice%20Bulletins/Committee%20on%20Practice%20 Bulletins%20Obstetrics/Screening%20for%20Fetal%20Aneuploidy.aspx. Published May 2016. Reaffirmed 2018.

OTHER TESTS IN OBSTETRICS AND GYNECOLOGY

BISHOP SCORING SYSTEM

- Indication: The Bishop scoring is used to evaluate the appropriateness of induction of labor.
  - Pertinent findings: Historically, a Bishop score higher than 8 in multiparous women with uncomplicated pregnancies and absence of contraindications was a good prognosticator for successful induction of labor (Table 4.16).
    - A simplified Bishop score[1] was developed in 2011, which only considered dilation, effacement, and station. A Bishop score higher than 5 was found to have equivalent positive predictive value to the original Bishop score of greater than 8.[1]

TABLE 4.16 Bishop Scoring System

Score	Dilation (cm)	Effacement (%)	Station	Cervical Consistency	Cervical Position
0	Closed	0–30	−3	Firm	Posterior
1	1–2	40–50	−2	Medium	Midposition
2	3–4	60–70	−1	Soft	Anterior
3	≥5	≥80	+1, +2		

> **CLINICAL PEARL:** Most providers will use the modified Bishop score in which dilation, effacement, and station are considered.

FERN TEST

Similar to the process used for nitrazine testing to aid in the diagnosis of rupture of membranes, a sterile speculum is inserted into the vagina, and, using a sterile swab, fluid from the posterior fornix is collected. The fluid is placed onto a slide, air dried, and then examined under a microscope.

- Indication: As an aid in the diagnosis of rupture of membranes
  - Pertinent findings: Amniotic fluid creates a fern-like pattern. The presence of pooling in the posterior fornix also aids in the diagnosis of rupture of membranes.

FETAL SCALP BLOOD

- Indication: During the intrapartum period, scalp blood sampling can be performed if the fetal heart rate pattern is nonreassuring. The fetal scalp is punctured and a small amount of blood is collected in a capillary tube. There are significant limitations to fetal scalp blood testing, including contamination with meconium or amniotic fluid.

- ○ Pertinent findings: A normal pH reassures that the fetus is not at immediate risk of hypoxia. If the pH is low, fetal acidosis is present and delivery should be expedited.

GENETIC TESTING: *BRCA,* LYNCH

The most commonly encountered genetic malignancies in OB/GYN are breast cancer, ovarian cancer, and uterine cancer. Appropriately identifying and stratifying patients and their risk is an important part of practice. The two most common syndromes associated with breast, ovarian, and uterine cancer are *BRCA* mutations and Lynch syndrome (hereditary nonpolyposis colorectal cancer). Peutz–Jeghers is a less commonly encountered syndrome that has associated breast, ovarian, colon, and gastrointestinal (GI) cancers. Cowden syndrome is another less commonly encountered syndrome that has associated breast, uterine, colon, and thyroid cancer.[2,3]

- Indication: To identify and stratify a woman's risk for hereditary cancer. ACOG recommends screening that includes a personal history of cancer, first- and second-degree family member history of cancer, and as much information as can be collected regarding age of onset, paternal versus maternal lineage, and the type of cancer.[2] Although some offices offer *BRCA1, BRCA2,* and Lynch syndrome testing, it is advised to refer women with a history suggestive of a hereditary cancer syndrome to a genetic counselor or other qualified healthcare provider for testing, patient education, and referrals.
  - ○ Clues to a possible genetic cancer syndrome include the following:
    - Young age at diagnosis
    - Multiple cancers in the same person or same organ
    - The same cancer in several generations along the same lineage (maternal or paternal)
    - Male breast cancer
    - Ashkenazi Jewish descent
    - Triple negative breast cancer
    - Epithelial ovarian, tubal, pancreatic, prostate, or peritoneal cancer
    - Colon cancer
    - Uterine cancer
    - Malignant melanoma
  - ○ Pertinent findings: The differences among *BRCA1, BRCA2,* and Lynch syndrome:
    - Women with the *BRCA1* mutation carry a 50% to 85% risk of developing breast cancer and a 40% to 60% chance of developing ovarian cancer. There is also an increased risk in developing a contralateral breast cancer.[3]

- Women with the *BRCA2* mutation also carry a 50% to 85% risk of developing breast cancer and a 16% to 27% risk of developing ovarian cancer. *BRCA2* mutation is also a risk factor for malignant melanoma and pancreatic cancer.[3]
- Women with Lynch syndrome carry a 52% to 82% risk of developing colorectal cancer, a 25% to 60% risk of developing uterine (endometrial) cancer, and a 4% to 24% risk of developing ovarian cancer.[1]
- However, hereditary breast cancer only accounts for up to 15% of all breast cancers, so a negative test can be falsely reassuring. In March 2018, the Food and Drug Administration (FDA) approved direct-to-consumer genetic testing and ACOG promptly replied with a statement outlining their concerns.[4]

ACOG recommends that women should only pursue this type of genetic testing under the care of a provider with experience and expertise in cancer genetics (e.g. a medical geneticist, genetic counselor, oncologist with expertise in cancer genetics, obstetrician–gynecologist with expertise in cancer genetics, or other similarly-qualified professionals). Should a patient pursue direct-to-consumer testing and seek medical advice after the results are available, the FDA recommends confirmatory testing and genetic counseling.

CLINICAL PEARL: Review the patient's medical and family history to assess candidacy for genetic testing. If there is a question about a possible hereditary cancer mutation, refer to a clinical geneticist.

GROUP B STREPTOCOCCUS/STREPTOCOCCUS AGALACTIAE[5]

Group *B Streptococcus* (GBS) is a common pathogen found in the vagina of women. It is considered nonpathogenic to the female. However, it is the leading cause of infection-related morbidity and mortality in newborns as it can cause sepsis, pneumonia, and meningitis.[5]

- Indication: Testing for GBS occurs via a rectovaginal swab collection in every gravid patient between 35 and 37 weeks' gestation. It is important to start the swabbing process at the introitus and move posteriorly to the rectum.
   - Pertinent findings: Women with GBS bacteriuria during the current pregnancy or who have a history of delivering a newborn with GBS disease do not need a repeat rectovaginal swab but will be managed with intrapartum antibiotics (see text that follows). When women present in labor with an unknown GBS result, GBS prophylaxis is advised if the patient has had an amniotic rupture for 18 hours or longer, fever greater than or equal to 100.4°F or 38.0°C; and is <37 weeks' gestation.

- Intrapartum treatment of GBS is with penicillin or ampicillin. Cefazolin can be used if the patient has a penicillin allergy, but only if anaphylaxis did not occur. If a patient is at high risk for developing anaphylaxis, the specimen can be sent for susceptibility to erythromycin and clindamycin. If there is a resistant organism, treatment with vancomycin is recommended. Use of erythromycin is not recommended due to high resistance rates.
- Doses of the recommended antibiotics:
  - Pen G: Five million units administered intravenously followed by 2.5 to 3 million units every 4 hours until delivery
  - Ampicillin: Two grams administered intravenously followed by 1 g every 4 hours until delivery
  - Cefazolin: Two grams administered intravenously followed by 1 g every 8 hours until delivery
  - Clindamycin: Administer 900 mg intravenously every 8 hours until delivery (use only if penicillin allergic and GBS is sensitive to clindamycin and erythromycin)
  - Vancomycin: Administer 1 g intravenously every 12 hours until delivery (use only if penicillin allergic and GBS is NOT sensitive to clindamycin and erythromycin)

NITRAZINE TEST

Nitrazine paper is used to aid in the diagnosis of several obstetrical and gynecological issues. For example, nitrazine paper is one way to screen for rupture of membranes. Insert a sterile speculum into the vagina. A sterile swab is used to collect fluid from the posterior fornix. Apply the fluid to a small piece of nitrazine, and if it turns blue, this is an indication of an alkaline pH.

- Indication: To test vaginal pH as an aid in the diagnosis of rupture of membranes or bacterial vaginosis
  - Pertinent findings: Nitrazine paper that turns blue indicates alkaline vaginal fluid. As amniotic fluid is alkaline, it can be helpful to rule out the presence of amniotic fluid if the paper stays yellow. However, blood, semen, and certain bacteria are alkalinic, so the nitrazine test is not diagnostic of rupture of membranes (see discussion of premature rupture of membranes for more information in Chapter 3, Common Disease Entities in Obstetrics).

UMBILICAL CORD BLOOD GAS

- Indication: Cord blood is obtained at the time of delivery and is a way to objectively assess the metabolic status of the newborn.
  - Pertinent findings: The arterial cord pH and base deficit calculation can identify perinatal hypoxia. A cord gas with a pH less than 7.0 and a base deficit greater than 12 mmol/L indicate fetal metabolic acidosis. Hypoxia and extent of fetal metabolic acidosis are correlated with poor fetal outcomes, including motor and cognitive deficits.

Zika Testing

- Indication: Both the Centers for Disease Control and Prevention (CDC) and ACOG provide guidance about Zika testing in women who are asymptomatic, at risk for developing Zika virus disease, pregnant, and considering pregnancy. During pregnancy, ACOG advises all women be asked whether they are at risk for exposure to Zika virus at each prenatal visit. Possible exposures include sex with a partner who resides in a geographic area at risk for Zika or who has traveled to an endemic area, and personal travel or residence in a geographic area at risk for Zika. The CDC and ACOG advised that women who are at risk of Zika virus disease or exposure should be offered a nucleic acid test (NAT). In the recent past, immunoglobulin M (IgM) testing was the only available serologic test, but IgM antibodies can persist for at least 4 months after exposure. Pregnant women at risk could be offered Zika NAT, dengue and Zika virus IgM, Zika virus plaque reduction neutralization test (PRNT), and dengue virus PRNT and IgM testing three times during pregnancy.[6,7]
  - ○ Pertinent findings: Zika virus can have devastating consequences to the fetus, including microcephaly and other brain anomalies. Zika disease can present with fever, rash, arthralgias, and conjunctivitis; some people have mild disease but can still carry the virus. Women who desire pregnancy should wait at least 8 weeks after possible exposure or symptom onset to attempt conception.
    - ■ If a pregnant woman has laboratory evidence of Zika virus, serial ultrasounds every 3 to 4 weeks should be administered to assess neuroanatomy and growth.

  For more details, see the CDC Zika virus testing algorithms:

  www.cdc.gov/mmwr/volumes/66/wr/mm6629e1.htm?s_cid=mm6629
  e1_w#F1_down

  www.cdc.gov/mmwr/volumes/66/wr/mm6629e1.htm?s_cid=mm6629
  e1_w#F2_down

References

1. Laughon SK, Zhang J, Troendle J, et al. Using a simplified Bishop score to predict vaginal delivery. *Obstet Gynecol*. 2011;117(4):805. doi:10.1097/AOG.0b013e3182114ad2

2. American College of Obstetricians and Gynecologists. Committee opinion no. 634. Hereditary cancer syndromes and risk assessment. https://www.acog.org/Clinical-Guidance-and-Publications/Committee-Opinions/Committee-on-Genetics/Hereditary-Cancer-Syndromes-and-Risk-Assessment. Accessed May 12, 2018.

3. American College of Obstetricians and Gynecologists. Practice advisory: response to FDA's authorization of *BRCA1 and BRCA2* gene mutation direct-to-consumer testing. https://www.acog.org/Clinical-Guidance-and-Publications/Practice-Advisories/Practice-Advisory-Response-to-FDAs-Authorization-of-BRCA1-and-BRCA2-Genes-Direct-to-Consumer-Testing. Accessed May 12, 2018.

4. Memorial Sloan Kettering Cancer Center. *BRCA1 and BRCA2* genes: risk for breast and ovarian cancer. https://www.mskcc.org/cancer-care/risk-assessment-screening/hereditary-genetics/genetic-counseling/brca1-brca2-genes-risk-breast-ovarian. Accessed May 12, 2018.

5. American College of Obstetricians and Gynecologists. Committee opinion no 782. Prevention of early-onset group B streptococcal disease in newborns. https://www.acog.org/Clinical-Guidance-and-Publications/Committee-Opinions/Committee-on-Obstetric-Practice/Prevention-of-Early-Onset-Group-B-Streptococcal-Disease-in-Newborns#here. Published June 25, 2019.

6. American College of Obstetricians and Gynecologists. Practice advisory interim guidance for care of obstetric patients during a Zika virus outbreak. https://www.acog.org/Clinical-Guidance-and-Publications/Practice-Advisories/Practice-Advisory-Interim-Guidance-for-Care-of-Obstetric-Patients-During-a-Zika-Virus-Outbreak#Figure%201%20sep%202017. Updated September 13, 2017.

7. Oduyebo T, Polen KD, Walke HT, et al. Update: interim guidance for health care providers caring for pregnant women with possible Zika virus exposure—United States (including U.S. territories). *MMWR Morb Mortal Wkly Rep.* 2017;66(29):781–793. doi:10.15585/mmwr.mm6629e1

5

Patient Education and Counseling in OB/GYN

BREASTFEEDING

ACOG recommends that women breastfeed for the first 6 months of the newborn's life. Start the discussion about breastfeeding early during pregnancy and offer support and education throughout the prenatal course. Women who want to breastfeed should be shown how and offered assistance during the first hour after delivery, if possible. Most hospitals offer lactation support specialists who can assist during the hospital stay and even be available once the patient is discharged to home. However, many women will call their OB/GYN provider with questions, so it is imperative that women are offered evidence-based helpful information to support breastfeeding. ACOG offers patient education and other materials at www.acog.org/About-ACOG/ACOG-Departments/Breastfeeding.

> **CLINICAL PEARL:** Breastfeeding is considered the optimal nutrition for newborns and infants through the first year of life. Preparation for breastfeeding should occur during pregnancy. Use your community resources, such as lactation consultants, if needed.

CONTRACEPTION

Issues and concerns regarding contraception are common reasons why women present to the clinic. There are many misconceptions regarding how contraceptives work, how to properly use them, and how to adjust if problems arise. You must familiarize yourself with all options and be able to advise women according to evidence-based guidelines.

One misconception is that a woman must have a Pap test or a pelvic examination before she can have her contraception either refilled or begun. Although Pap testing certainly reduces the overall incidence of cervical cancer, it is not appropriate to withhold contraception because a woman is late for her Pap test. A reminder that she needs a Pap is appropriate, as is allowing her a few months to come in. If a patient has a history of abnormal Pap screening and needs a colposcopy or a follow-up Pap, it is still not appropriate to withhold contraception. Provide written and verbal documentation of the necessity of either rescreening with Pap or colposcopy and that the patient was advised that no further refills will be given if she does not return for whichever test she needs by the given timeline.

Combined oral contraceptive pills (COCPs). COCPs are about 91% effective[1] but this percentage can be higher with perfect use. These pills contain estradiol and progestin. It is important to screen for contraindications before prescribing COCPs (see Tables 5.1 and 5.2). COCPs have short half-lives, so pills must be taken every day at the same time. If a patient misses one pill, she can double up the next day. If a patient misses two pills in a row, she can double her pills for the next 2 days, but must use a back-up method such as condoms or abstinence.

The only antimicrobial associated with decreased contraceptive pill efficacy is rifampin.[2] However, patients who are taking antiepileptic medications, such as carbamazepine, phenytoin, primidone, topiramate, barbiturates, or oxcarbazepine, should not use estrogen-containing contraception as they compete for hepatic clearance and the seizure threshold will be lowered.

The different types of COCPs depend on the estrogen and progestin dosage and whether the dosages change during the pill pack.

- Monophasic pills: The same dose of estrogen and progestin throughout the pill pack
- Multiphasic pills: The dosage of estrogen and progestin changes during the pill pack; pills vary among two different dosages (biphasic), three different dosages (triphasic), to four different dosages (four-phase)
- Some pill packs will have a full 7 days of placebo; others include from two to four placebo pills
- Ethinyl estradiol is the synthetic estrogen used in almost all pills in the United States
  - Most pills are now 10 to 20 mcg and are referred to as *low dose.*
  - Pills that are 30 to 35 mcg are considered middle dose.
  - Pills with 50 mcg are considered high dose.
    - High-dose pills are more closely associated with adverse thromboembolic events and should be avoided.
- Progestins are classified by their androgenicity.
  - Norgestrel and levonorgestrel are highly androgenic.

○ Norethindrone acetate, desogestrel, and norgestimate are weakly androgenic.
○ Drospirenone is antiandrogenic.

Patch. This is about 91% effective.[1] Does not protect against sexually transmitted infections (STIs). Contains estrogen and a progestin.

- The patch is replaced every week for 3 weeks followed by 1 week without a patch.
- Effectiveness is decreased in women with higher body mass indices (BMIs).

Monthly vaginal ring. Rings are about 91% effective.[1] Does not protect against STIs. Contains estrogen and a progestin.

- Contains etonogestrel and ethinyl estradiol.
- The flexible ring is inserted into the vagina and left in place for 3 weeks.
- The package insert recommends the woman go 1 week without the ring.

Annual vaginal ring. This is about 96% effective.[1] It does not protect against STIs. Contains estrogen and a progestin.

- A flexible ring with segesterone acetate and ethinyl estradiol
- The ring is inserted into the vagina and left in place for 3 weeks
- The package insert recommends removal for 1 week to allow for a withdrawal bleed
- During the week the ring is out, it is appropriately washed and kept in its case
- The annual ring does not need to be refrigerated

Intrauterine system (IUS). Considered an LARC; an IUS is more than 99% effective.[1] It does not protect against STIs.

- Progestin-secreting IUSs can reduce menstrual bleeding.
- Copper IUSs can be used in women with contraindications to estrogen (Table 5.1) and progestin (Table 5.2) but can cause heavier vaginal bleeding.
- ACOG guidelines do not mandate a woman be tested for STIs prior to an IUS insertion. You may screen for STIs at the time of insertion, and, if they come back positive, you can treat. Women may end up with an unplanned conception due to the delay if you check STIs first.
- LARCs are appropriate immediately postpartum, at the 4- to 6-week postpartum visit, in nulliparous women, and in adolescents.
- Copper IUSs can be used as an emergency contraceptive.

Progestin-only pills. These pills are about 97% effective[3] with perfect use. They do not protect against STIs.

- Progestin-only pills are appropriate for breastfeeding women and women with contraindications to estrogen use, but make sure patients

TABLE 5.1 Contraindications for Estrogen

History of or current breast cancer
Coronary heart disease (CHD)
Previous venous thromboembolic event or stroke
Active liver disease
Unexplained vaginal bleeding
High-risk endometrial cancer
Transient ischemic attack

TABLE 5.2 Contraindications for Progestin

Current or past history of thrombophlebitis or thromboembolic disorders
Liver dysfunction or disease
Known or suspected malignancy of breast or genital organs
Undiagnosed vaginal bleeding
Pregnancy

do not have a contraindication to progestin use as well. Due to the short half-life, they must be taken every day at the same time.

- There are no placebo pills in progestin-only pill packs.

Progestin injection (depot-medroxyprogesterone acetate [DMPA]). Injections are about 94% effective.[1] They do not protect against STIs.

- Administered intramuscularly every 12 to 13 weeks so patient must come back to the office for repeat injections.
- Long-term use of DMPA is associated with a loss of bone mineral density.[4]

Subdermal implant. Implants are about 99% effective.[1] They do not protect against STIs.

- This is a progestin-only secreting device that is placed in the nondominant upper inner arm and is good for up to 3 years.

Sponge. Sponges are up to 88% effective[1] with perfect use. They do not protect against STIs.

Diaphragm. The diaphragm is about 88% effective.[1] It does not protect against STIs.

Condoms. Condoms are about 82% effective.[1] When used with other modalities, their effectiveness is increased and condoms helps prevent certain STIs.

Spermicide. Spermicide is about 70% effective.[1] It does not protect against STIs.

Tubal ligation. This procedure is about 99% effective.[1] It does not protect against STIs.

Fertility awareness. This is up to 86% effective.[1] It does not protect against STIs.

Breastfeeding. Can be highly effective when the patient is not supplementing with formula. Does not protect against STIs.

- Should be used as short-term contraception only.[1]

Withdrawal. This is up to 78% effective.[1] It does not protect against STIs.

> **CLINICAL PEARL:** A careful history can uncover a patient's potential contraindication or precaution to estrogen or progestin use. Also remember to provide patient education on all of the options so that the patient can make the best choice for herself and her reproductive goals.

REFERENCES

1. Centers for Disease Control and Prevention. Effectiveness of family planning methods. https://www.cdc.gov/reproductivehealth/contraception/unintendedpreg nancy/pdf/Contraceptive_methods_508.pdf. Published August 14, 3013. Updated August 29, 2013.
2. Simmons KB, Haddad LB, Nanda K, Curtis KM. Drug interactions between nonrifamycin antibiotics and hormonal contraception: a systematic review. *Am J Obstet Gynecol.* 2018;218(1):88–97. doi:10.1016/j.ajog.2017.07.003
3. Centers for Disease Control and Prevention. US selected practice recommendations for contraceptive use, 2016: progestin-only pills. https://www.cdc .gov/reproductivehealth/contraception/mmwr/spr/progestin.html
4. Beksinska ME, Smit JA. Hormonal contraception and bone mineral density. *Expert Rev Obstet Gynecol.* 2011;6(3):305–319. doi:10.1586/eog.11.19

IMMUNIZATIONS IN PREGNANCY

ACOG recommends that all women who are pregnant or will be pregnant during the influenza season receive an inactivated influenza vaccine. Varicella and MMR are contraindicated in pregnancy. Tdap (tetanus, diphtheria, and pertussis) is recommended between 27 and 36 weeks' gestation in each pregnancy. HPV vaccination should be avoided during pregnancy. Hepatitis A, hepatitis B, rabies, meningococcal and pneumococcal vaccination can be given in select populations depending on risk factors. Postpartum vaccinations include MMR, varicella, Tdap if the patient did not receive it during pregnancy, and HPV.[1]

Hepatitis B vaccination is indicated in pregnant patients in the following circumstances:

- In order to complete the Hepatitis B series if initiated before conception
- Women who are unvaccinated and at high risk for hepatitis B infection

CLINICAL PEARL: HPV vaccination is indicated up to age 45 years, but check the patient's insurance coverage prior to administering the vaccine to ensure coverage.

REFERENCE

1. American College of Obstetricians and Gynecologists. Committee opinion no. 741. Maternal immunization. https://www.acog.org/Clinical-Guidance-and-Publications/Committee-Opinions/Immunization-Infectious-Disease-and-Public-Health-Preparedness-Expert-Work-Group/Maternal-Immunization. Published June 2018.

IMMUNIZATIONS IN THE NONPREGNANT WOMAN

ACOG supports the Advisory Committee on Immunization Practices (ACIP) and CDC recommendations regarding immunization. Discussions about immunization status are appropriate during routine health maintenance visits and during pregnancy. The HPV vaccine should be initiated when the patient is 11 or 12 years, but if the patient has not yet received the vaccine, she can still begin up until age 26 years. Other important vaccines include Tdap, measles, mumps, and rubella (MMR), varicella, hepatitis B, meningococcus, and pneumococcus. Hepatitis A can be administered in at-risk patients.

INTIMATE PARTNER VIOLENCE

Intimate partner violence (IPV) can affect any woman, regardless of ethnicity, race, religion, socioeconomic status, and sexual orientation. IPV can contribute to unintended pregnancy, STIs, and pregnancy complications. ACOG recommends screening all women for IPV at each health visit and as a routine part of prenatal care. The following should guide IPV screening:[1]

- Ask about IPV when the woman is alone.
- Do not use family or friends as interpreters.
- Reinforce that all women are screened for IPV and that confidentiality is upheld.
- Know your community resources so that appropriate and timely referrals can be made.
- Printed patient education materials with hotlines and other information should be easily accessible.
- Training of staff and other healthcare providers should be offered.

One suggestion for how to ask about IPV is to use the SAFE questions.[2]

S: Stress/safety—Do you feel safe or stressed in your relationship?

A: Afraid/abused—Are you now, or have you been, in a relationship where you feel afraid or suffered abuse?

F: Friends/family—Are your friends aware of your current situation and that you are/may be hurt?

E: Emergency plan—Do you have a safe place to go if you need to leave?

CLINICAL PEARL: Know the domestic violence/IPV resources available in your area and be ready to contact the appropriate agencies when necessary.

REFERENCES

1. The American College of Obstetricians and Gynecologists. Committee opinion no. 518. Intimate partner violence. https://www.acog.org/Clinical-Guidance-and-Publications/Committee-Opinions/Committee-on-Health-Care-for-Underserved-Women/Intimate-Partner-Violence. Published February 2012. Reaffirmed 2019.

2. Ashur ML. Asking about domestic violence: SAFE questions. *JAMA*. 1993; 269(18):2367. doi:10.1001/jama.1993.03500180059027

KEGELS

Kegel exercises can help prevent pelvic floor laxity. Pelvic floor laxity is associated with pelvic organ prolapse and urinary incontinence.

There are two layers of the pelvic floor musculature. The superficial layer consists of the bulbocavernosus, the ischiocavernosus, the superficial transverse perineal, and the external anal sphincter. The deep layer includes the deep transverse perineal, the compressor urethra, and the uretrovaginal sphincter. Both the superficial and deep layers are innervated by the pudendal nerve. The pelvic diaphragm consists of the levator ani, which includes the pubococcygeus and iliococcygeus, the piriformis, and the obturator internus. The way to identify the correct muscles used for Kegel exercises is to try and stop urination. Many women incorrectly perform Kegels by contracting the gluteals and although that may increase muscle tone in the buttocks, it will not help strengthen the pelvic floor. The idea is to identify the proper muscle group, hold for 5 seconds, and release. Once the patient is confident of the identification of the correct muscles, she can increase the hold to 10 seconds. Tell your patient to perform Kegels often throughout the day. Some women will even perform Kegels during sexual intercourse.

> **CLINICAL PEARL:** If the patient is having a difficult time isolating the proper muscles, refer to a physical therapist who specializes in women's health.

MAMMOGRAPHY

Various professional organizations have attempted to develop consensus guidelines regarding mammography. ACOG revised its mammography guidelines to include the importance of shared decision-making between provider and patient regarding screening initiation, frequency, and termination of screening.[1]

ACOG recommends the following:

- Ages 40 to 44: Women should have the choice to begin mammographic screening
- Ages 45 to 54: Women should have screening mammograms annually, but can defer to every 2 years
- Ages 55+: Women should have screening mammography every 2 years, but can opt for annual screening
- If women have not begun screening in their 40s, screening should begin no later than 50 years.
- Mammography should be done every year or every 2 years based on the patient's preferences and an open discussion regarding the risks and benefits of screening at different intervals.
- Mammography should continue until age 75 years. After 75 years, a discussion regarding the risks and benefits of continued mammography should be initiated and the decision to continue based on shared decision-making. If the patient is in otherwise good health and has a life expectancy of at least 10 years, screening should continue.

> **CLINICAL PEARL:** Deciding on a screening strategy should be a shared decision between the provider and the patient with careful attention paid to the patient's risk factors, goals, and current state of the evidence.

REFERENCE

1. American College of Obstetricians and Gynecologists. ACOG revises breast cancer screening guidance: ob-gyns promote shared decision making. https://www.acog.org/About-ACOG/News-Room/News-Releases/2017/ACOG-Revises-Breast-Cancer-Screening-Guidance--ObGyns-Promote-Shared-Decision-Making. Published June 22, 2017.

Pap/Human Papillomavirus Testing

Pap testing to screen for cervical cancer should begin at age 21 years in average risk women* unless the patient has HIV or immunocompromised from other disorders. The following guidelines apply to women who are not HIV+, immunocompromised, have a history of cervical cancer, or a daughter of a woman who used diethylstilbestrol (DES).[1]

- *Age 21 to 29 years:* Cervical cytology alone every 3 years. Routine human papillomavirus (HPV) cotesting is not recommended
- HPV screening without cytology can be used in women 25 years and older if they are HIV negative and not otherwise immunocompromised*
- *Age 30 to 65 years:* Cotesting with HPV and cytology every 5 years or cytology alone every 3 years
- *Age 65+ years:* Screening should be discontinued if there is evidence of adequate screening with negative results (three consecutive negative screenings with cytology alone or two consecutive negative screenings with cotesting within the past 10 years, so long as the most recent screening was within the past 5 years); and no prior history of cervical intraepithelial lesion (CIN) 2 or higher

*Women who have a history of CIN 2 or 3 or adenocarcinoma in situ should be screened for 20 years even if it means extending screening past 65 years. In women with risk factors, screening may occur at more frequent intervals. Risk factors include the following: HIV+, immunocompromise, exposure to diethylstilbestrol, history of CIN 2 or 3 or cancer.

Reference

1. American College of Obstetricians and Gynecologists. ACOG practice bulletin No. 168. Cervical cancer screening and prevention. Interim update. https://www.acog.org/Clinical%20Guidance%20and%20Publications/Practice%20Bulletins/Committee%20on%20Practice%20Bulletins%20Gynecology/Cervical%20Cancer%20Screening%20and%20Prevention.aspx. Published October 2016. Reaffirmed 2018.

Patient Education During Pregnancy

All pregnant women should engage in some sort of aerobic exercise during pregnancy but must be cautious when beginning a new exercise regimen during pregnancy. Encourage your patients to take regular brisk walks.

- Relative contraindications to aerobic exercise during pregnancy include the following:
  - Any cardiac arrhythmia that has not undergone cardiac evaluation
  - Maternal anemia
  - Intrauterine growth restriction
  - Morbid obesity (particularly if the patient has not previously exercised)
  - Body mass index (BMI) less than 12
  - Poorly controlled diabetes, hypertension, seizure disorder, or pulmonary disease
  - Orthopedic or musculoskeletal limitations

- Absolute contraindications to aerobic exercise during pregnancy include the following:
  - Heart disease that results in hemodynamic compromise
  - Restrictive lung disease
  - Bleeding during the second or third trimester
  - Cervical insufficiency
  - Placental previa (after 26 weeks)
  - Preterm labor and preterm rupture of membranes
  - Preeclampsia

- First-trimester considerations
  - Review of prenatal visit schedule, ultrasound recommendations, fetal aneuploidy testing
  - Ancillary testing
  - Zika exposure assessment
  - Depression screen
  - Illicit drugs, alcohol, and tobacco use
  - Intimate partner violence
  - Psychosocial barriers to care, safe housing, communication barriers, work hazards
  - Nutrition counseling, including appropriate weight gain during pregnancy and Women, Infants, and Children (WIC) referral if needed
  - Toxoplasmosis avoidance (cat litter, raw meat)
  - Medication use, including over-the-counter medications and dietary supplements
  - Oral health, including referral to dentist if appropriate
  - Exercise (see earlier text)
  - Sexual activity
  - Avoidance of saunas and hot tubs
  - Seat belt and helmet use
  - Information on hospital of delivery
  - Childbirth classes
  - Barriers to breastfeeding

- Second-trimester considerations
  - Zika testing if necessary
  - Review of signs and symptoms of preterm labor

- Pediatrician selection (if not already established)
- Postpartum contraception and planning (the idea is to begin the discussion)
- Reassess tobacco, alcohol, and drug use
- Depression screen (if not already completed and as appropriate)
- Intimate partner violence

- Third-trimester considerations
  - Zika testing if necessary
  - Fetal movement/fetal kick counts
  - Signs and symptoms of preeclampsia
  - Signs of labor, when to call the office, when to go to the hospital
  - Braxton Hicks contractions
  - Childbirth-specific counseling: Trial of labor after cesarean (TOLAC), labor expectations, pain control, when to go to the hospital, when to call the office, who will be present to support the patient
  - Postpartum contraception (e.g., immediate long-acting reversible contraceptive [LARC])
  - Breastfeeding: Support offered, prescription for breast pump and supplies if needed
  - Family Medical Leave Act (FMLA) and disability paperwork/plans
  - Depression screening/postpartum depression
  - Alcohol, tobacco, and drug use
  - Intimate partner violence
  - Child safety seat

- Postpartum
  - Infant feeding
  - Postpartum depression
  - Lochia
  - Wound healing (postepisiotomy, lacerations, or cesarean incision)
  - Sex after baby
  - Contraception
  - Breastfeeding
  - Emotional changes
  - Hair loss
  - Follow-up for preeclampsia/eclampsia/gestational hypertension (HTN; see "Gestational Hypertension" in Chapter 3, Common Disease Entities: Obstetrics)
  - Follow-up for gestational diabetes (see "Gestational Diabetes Mellitus" section in Chapter 3, Common Disease Entities in Obstetrics)

CLINICAL PEARL: Most nulligravida patients will require extra time at each visit for questions. Each prenatal visit is a tremendous opportunity to provide patient education so take the extra time and enjoy the dialogue.

Peri- and Postmenopausal Health

Bone health. Women 19 to 50 years should have at least 1,000 mg of calcium and 600 mg of vitamin D every day. Women 51 to 70 should have 1,200 mg of calcium and 600 mg of vitamin D each day, and women 71 years and older should continue 1,200 mg of daily calcium but increase their vitamin D to 800 mg. Screening for osteoporosis with DEXA scanning should begin at 65 years unless the patient has risk factors for osteoporosis, including a personal history of a fragility fracture, rheumatoid arthritis, tobacco use, alcoholism, or other medical or pharmacologic causes of accelerated bone loss.

Heart health. Screening with EKG, coronary calcium, or other biomarkers in otherwise low-risk women is not recommended. Maintaining an active healthy lifestyle, not using tobacco, and limiting alcohol intake is important throughout the life span. Estrogen, although it may intrinsically be cardio-protective, is not recommended for prevention of cardiovascular disease.

Mammography. See "Mammography" section previously in this chapter.

Colonoscopy.[1] The U.S. Preventive Services Taskforce recommends screening at age 50 in average risk patients, and screening should cease at 75 years. Available modalities include fecal immunochemical tests (FITs), flexible sigmoidoscopy, and guaiac-based fecal occult blood tests (gFOBT), although FITs have increased sensitivity over gFOBT.

Reference

1. U.S. Preventive Services Task Force. Final recommendation statement: colorectal cancer: screening. 2016. https://www.uspreventiveservicestaskforce.org/Page/Document/RecommendationStatementFinal/colorectal-cancer-screening2#tab

Postmenopausal Hormone Use

ACOG and the North American Menopause Society (NAMS) do not recommend hormone use for the prevention of cardiovascular disease or Alzheimer's dementia.[1] ACOG and NAMS do recommend the lowest dose of systemic estrogen for vasomotor symptoms association with menopause. In patients with the genitourinary syndrome of menopause and no or minimal vasomotor symptoms, the recommendation is vaginal estradiol or vaginal dehydroepiandrosterone (DHEA). Women with a uterus who use vaginal estrogen do not need a progestin. Systemic estrogen helps prevent bone loss and osteoporosis and is the best choice for women younger than 60 years. The lowest dose estrogen patch (0.014 mg/d) currently available is indicated for prevention of osteoporosis but may not alleviate vasomotor symptoms. Another option to help prevent bone loss is a selective estrogen receptor modulator.[1,2]

In women who still have a uterus, the addition of a progestin to systemic estrogen is essential to protect the endometrium from endometrial hyperplasia and cancer.

> **CLINICAL PEARL:** Shared decision-making involving the risks, benefits, and alternatives to postmenopausal hormone use is critical, as is documentation of the conversation and the patient's goals.

REFERENCES

1. American College of Obstetricians and Gynecologists. Committee opinion no. 565. Hormone therapy and heart disease. https://www.acog.org/Clinical-Guidance-and-Publications/Committee-Opinions/Committee-on-Gynecologic-Practice/Hormone-Therapy-and-Heart-Disease. Published June 2013. Reaffirmed 2018.
2. The NAMS Hormone Therapy Position Statement Advisory Panel. The 2017 hormone therapy position statement of the North American Menopause Society. *Menopause.* 2017;24(7):728–753. doi:10.1097/GME.0000000000000921

REPRODUCTIVE HEALTH

Essential questions to ask women of reproductive age (who still have a uterus):[1]

1. Do you have a desire to become pregnant within the next year?
    a. If the answer is no, discuss contraceptive options and safe sex practices.
    b. If the answer is yes, discuss procreative counseling.
2. Do you want to have more children, and, if so, about how many and in what time frame?

Procreative counseling should include the following: assessing risk for sexually transmitted infections (STIs); immunization status; substance abuse; screening for interpersonal violence; medical/surgical/psychiatric history; review of medications that may be teratogenic or not recommended in pregnancy; maternal and paternal genetic history; body weight and nutritional status; environmental exposures to potentially toxic or harmful chemicals; and assessment of educational, socioeconomic, and cultural status so that patient education will be appropriate and meaningful.

Safe-sex practices. Patient education on safe sex is imperative. Remind all women who are sexually active that use of condoms and dental dams can help prevent some STIs, but that the risk of anorectal and oropharyngeal cancers due to human papillomavirus (HPV) is still present.

Contraceptive options. All women who do not desire pregnancy should be counseled on contraceptive options. Providing accurate and evidence-based information regarding all options is our obligation as physician assistants (PAs; see the "Contraception" section).

Kegels. Kegel exercises can help maintain the integrity of the pelvic floor muscles, reducing the risk of pelvic organ prolapse and urinary incontinence. See discussion on Kegels previously in this chapter.

Pap and STI screening. For women 21 years and older, discuss Papanicolaou testing guidelines and STI screening. If your patient is not yet due for a Pap test, discuss STI risk and test accordingly. Also remember that the U.S. Preventive Services Taskforce (USPSTF) recommends screening all adults who were born between 1945 and 1965 for Hepatitis C one time.[2] The USPSTF also recommends screening for HIV between the ages of 15 and 65 years, and in all pregnant women.[3]

Lesbian, gay, bisexual, and transgender (LGBT) issues.[4] Lesbian and bisexual women may have concerns regarding disclosing their sexual orientation to healthcare providers and thus may experience barriers to healthcare. Women who have sex with women, who identify as either lesbian or bisexual, still need Pap testing. There are indicators that women in lesbian relationships are at greater risk for intimate partner violence so appropriate screening is recommended. Transgender issues are becoming more common and these patients may present at the OB/GYN office. Always be cognizant of the mental health issues that may accompany transgender patients, particularly during adolescence. Transgender males, when early in the transition process, may still have ovaries and a uterus so these patients need appropriate health maintenance during (and even after) their transition. In addition, the rate of suicide attempts among transgender individuals is about 40%, much higher than the national average of 4% among nontransgender individuals.[5]

Breast health. American College of Obstetricians and Gynecologists (ACOG) recommends that women 40 years and older receive an annual clinical breast exam. It is important to discuss with your patients the current mammography recommendations, self-breast examination techniques and limitations, and their overall risk for breast cancer. ACOG supports shared decision-making regarding the risks and benefits of mammography, when to begin screening, and screening intervals.[6]

Bone health.[7] Bone mass peaks around age 19 years and begins to rapidly decline around menopause. Women who have anorexia nervosa, use synthetic progestins long term (e.g., depot-medroxyprogesterone acetate), and take aromatase inhibitors are at greater risk for developing osteopenia and osteoporosis. Ways to improve bone health include adequate amounts of vitamin D and calcium, weight-bearing exercises, not smoking tobacco, and limiting alcohol intake.

- Women 19 to 50 years should have at least 1,000 mg of calcium and 600 mg of vitamin D every day.
- Women 51 to 70 should have 1,200 mg of calcium and 600 mg of vitamin D each day.
- Women 71 years and older should continue 1,200 mg of daily calcium but increase their vitamin D to 800 mg.
- Screening for osteoporosis with dual energy x-ray absorptiometry (DEXA) scanning should begin at 65 years unless the patient has risk factors for osteoporosis, including a personal history of a fragility fracture, rheumatoid arthritis, tobacco use, alcoholism, or other medical or pharmacologic causes of accelerated bone loss.[7]

CLINICAL PEARL: One of the most important activities in the practice of OB/GYN is engaging in meaningful patient education. Know where you can find resources. ACOG publishes appropriate patient education brochures on most topics encountered in an OB/GYN practice.

REFERENCES

1. American College of Obstetricians and Gynecologists. Committee opinion no. 654. Reproductive life planning to reduce unintended pregnancy. *Obstet Gynecol.* 2016;127:e66–e69. doi:10.1097/AOG.0000000000001314
2. U.S. Preventive Services Task Force. Hepatitis C: screening. https://www.us preventiveservicestaskforce.org/Page/Document/UpdateSummaryFinal/hepatitis -c-screening. Published June 2013.
3. U.S. Preventive Services Task Force. Human immunodeficiency virus (HIV) infection: screening. https://www.uspreventiveservicestaskforce.org/Page/Document/UpdateSummaryFinal/human-immunodeficiency-virus-hiv-infection-screening. Published April 2013.
4. American College of Obstetricians and Gynecologists. Health care for lesbians and bisexual women. Committee opinion no. 525. https://www.acog.org/Clinical -Guidance-and-Publications/Committee-Opinions/Committee-on-Health-Care -for-Underserved-Women/Health-Care-for-Lesbians-and-Bisexual-Women. Published May 2012. Reaffirmed 2018.
5. Haas AP, Rodgers PL, Herman JL. Suicide attempts among transgender and gender non-conforming adults: findings of the National Transgender Discrimination Survey. https://williamsinstitute.law.ucla.edu/wp-content/uploads/AFSP -Williams-Suicide-Report-Final.pdf. Published January 2014.
6. American College of Obstetricians and Gynecologists. ACOG revises breast cancer screening guidance: ob-gyns promote shared decision making. https://www.acog.org/About-ACOG/News-Room/News-Releases/2017/ACOG -Revises-Breast-Cancer-Screening-Guidance--ObGyns-Promote-Shared-Decision -Making?IsMobileSet=false. Published June 22, 2017.
7. American College of Obstetricians and Gynecologists. Practice bulletin no. 129. Osteoporosis. https://www.acog.org/Clinical%20Guidance%20and%20Publications/Practice%20Bulletins/Committee%20on%20Practice%20Bulletins%20Gynecology/Osteoporosis.aspx. Published September 2012. Reaffirmed 2019.

6

Urgent Management of OB/GYN Conditions

Introduction

The following sections describe some of the more common urgent conditions you may encounter in your OB/GYN clinical rotation. Please note that protocols may vary depending upon your facility and preceptor.

ACUTE SEVERE UTERINE BLEEDING (MENORRHAGIA)

Overview and Presentation

- Abnormal uterine bleeding can result in acute blood loss that causes hemodynamic compromise, so prompt evaluation of vital signs is important.[1]
- Acute abnormal bleeding can occur as a single episode or in a patient with a history of abnormal uterine bleeding.
- The history should focus on duration of bleeding and a quantification of bleeding typically by how many pads and/or tampons are being used and how frequently the patient is changing them.
- A careful physical examination must include a pelvic exam to locate the source of bleeding.
- Using the PALM-COEIN system can help to direct the history and physical examination to rule in or rule out the most common etiologies.

  P: Polyps
  A: Adenomyosis
  L: Leiomyoma

M: Malignancy
C: Coagulopathy
O: Ovulatory dysfunction
E: Endometrial
I: Iatrogenic
N: Not otherwise classified

Diagnostic Evaluation

- Women with abnormal uterine bleeding who have had consistent heavy menses since menarche, abnormal surgical or dental bleeding, postpartum hemorrhage, unexplained epistaxis or bruising, and/or a family history of a blood dyscrasia should be evaluated for a platelet or coagulation disorder.
- Young women, particularly adolescents with acute severe uterine bleeding, should be evaluated for Von Willebrand's disease.
- Laboratory tests must include a complete blood count (CBC) with differential, a serum beta-HCG, and type and cross.
- Laboratory tests for hemostatic disorders include partial thromboplastin time (PTT), activated partial thromboplastin time (aPTT), and fibrinogen.
- Laboratory tests for Von Willebrand disease include von Willebrand factor (VWF) antigen.

Management

- Urgent management includes pharmacologic and surgical modalities.
- Pharmacologic interventions include conjugated equine estrogen 25 mg intravenously every 4 to 6 hours for a maximum of 24 hours in the absence of contraindications.
- Medroxyprogesterone acetate 20 mg orally three times a day for 7 days can be used if the patient cannot use estrogen but has no contraindications to progestins.
  - Use of tranexamic acid is an important component of managing acute hemorrhage.
  - Tranexamic acid 1.3 g orally or 10 mg/kg intravenously for a maximum of 600 mg every 8 hours for 5 days is a nonhormonal option.
  - Tranexamic acid should not be used in patients with a history of a thrombotic or thromboembolic event and used with caution in patients who are currently taking combined oral contraceptive pills.
- Patients should be evaluated for transfusion per the institution's protocol.
- Combined hormonal contraception can be used for prevention of further bleeding episodes in the absence of contraindications.
- Other options for urgent control of uterine bleeding include dilation and curettage, uterine artery embolization, uterine tamponade, and hysterectomy.
- Endometrial ablation and insertion of a progestin-secreting intrauterine system (IUS) can also help prevent further episodes of bleeding.

> **CLINICAL PEARL:** Remember that in a patient with acute bleeding, you may not immediately see a decrease in the hemoglobin and hematocrit.

REFERENCE

1. American College of Obstetricians and Gynecologists. Committee opinion no. 557. Management of acute abnormal uterine bleeding in nonpregnant reproductive-aged women. https://www.acog.org/Clinical-Guidance-and-Publications/Committee-Opinions/Committee-on-Gynecologic-Practice/Management-of-Acute-Abnormal-Uterine-Bleeding-in-Nonpregnant-Reproductive-Aged-Women. Published April 2013. Reaffirmed 2019.

ACUTE UTERINE INVERSION

Overview and Presentation

- Uterine inversion will appear as a bleeding mass at the introitus after a vaginal delivery.[1,2]
- Uterine inversion is caused by a manual pulling force on the umbilical cord during delivery of the placenta.
- Inversion can also occur with a short umbilical cord, excessive fundal pressure, or rapid removal of the placenta.
- Massive hemorrhage and pain will be present.

Diagnostic Evaluation

- There are no diagnostic tests recommended for an acute uterine inversion.
- The diagnosis is a clinical one.

Management

- Manual replacement of the uterus should be attempted but may require the use of anesthesia, tocolysis, and pitocin as uterine inversion is strongly associated with postpartum hemorrhage.
- Manual replacement involves using the palm or fist of one hand and placing upward pressure with the fingers.
- In refractory cases, hysterectomy may be required.

REFERENCES

1. Avery DM. Obstetric emergencies. *Am J Clin Med.* 2009;6(2):42–47. https://www.aapsus.org/wp-content/uploads/Obstetric-Emergencies.pdf
2. American College of Obstetricians and Gynecologists. Practice bulletin no. 183. Postpartum hemorrhage. https://www.acog.org/Clinical-Guidance-and-Publications/Practice-Bulletins/Committee-on-Practice-Bulletins-Obstetrics/Postpartum-Hemorrhage. Accessed May 29, 2018.

AMNIOTIC FLUID EMBOLISM

Overview and Presentation[1,2]

- Although rare, amniotic fluid embolism (AFE) can be fatal, with mortality rates reportedly as high as 90%.[1,2]
- If women survive, common sequelae include neurologic impairment, renal failure, and heart failure.
- Women with an AFE typically present with acute respiratory distress after pushing during delivery or immediately after the delivery.
- Early signs include cough, altered mental status, cyanosis and hypoxia, fetal bradycardia and hypoxia, and hypotension.
- An AFE causes pulmonary vascular obstruction, pulmonary hypertension, cor pulmonale and left ventricular failure, shock, hypoxia, and DIC/hemorrhage.
- The following must be present to diagnose AFE:
  - Cardiac arrest or hypotension
  - Acute hypoxia
  - Severe hemorrhage or coagulopathy when other etiologies have been ruled out
  - The preceding occur during labor and delivery, cesarean, dilation and evacuation, or within 30 minutes' postpartum, when other etiologies have been ruled out

Diagnostic Evaluation

- There are no approved laboratory tests for the diagnosis of AFE, although numerous markers of inflammation are currently being studied.

Management

- Immediate management of the patient with an AFE includes immediate cardiopulmonary resuscitative measures.
- Mechanical ventilation and other critical care measures may be initiated, including inotropic support and vasopressors.
- Blood transfusion and correction of coagulopathy will be initiated.
- If the patient has not yet delivered, an emergency cesarean will be performed as fetal survival depends on rapid delivery within 5 minutes of cardiovascular collapse.

> **CLINICAL PEARL:** An AFE requires a rapid response. Review advanced cardiac life support (ACLS) protocols prior to your OB/GYN rotation.

References

1. Avery DM. Obstetric emergencies. *Am J Clin Med.* 2009;6(2):42–47. https://www.aapsus.org/wp-content/uploads/Obstetric-Emergencies.pdf
2. Kaur K, Bhardwaj M, Kumar P, et al. Amniotic fluid embolism. *J Anaethesiol Clin Pharmacol.* 2016;32(2):153–159. doi:10.4103/0970-9185.173356

Hyperemesis Gravidarum

Overview and Presentation

- Although death from nausea and vomiting in pregnancy is exceedingly rare, hyperemesis gravadarum (HG) can cause significant distress to the pregnant patient.[1]
- HG that results in dehydration can cause acute renal injury, esophageal tears, and Wernicke's encephalopathy.
- Patients with HG have persistent, unremitting episodes of nausea and vomiting despite conservative measures to treat.

Diagnostic Evaluation

- The diagnosis of HG is typically one of exclusion.
- The presence of ketonuria and weight loss (usually defined as a loss of 5% of pre pregnancy body weight) in the absence of other disorders is typically sufficient for the diagnosis.

Management

- Management of HG should actually begin when the patient first presents with nausea and vomiting, prior to developing HG.
- Nonpharmacologic options include ginger and acupressure, although the evidence to support either is lacking.
- Initial pharmacologic options include vitamin B6 and doxylamine, now available as a prescription in combined form.
- If B6 and doxylamine do not control nausea and vomiting, promethazine or dimenhydrinate can be prescribed, but caution is advised as both of these products cause somnolence.
- Once the patient progresses to HG and dehydration is present, fluid support as well as a pharmacologic intervention are needed.
- Normal saline is often the fluid of choice, but consider a dextrose formulation if the patient cannot tolerate anything PO (by mouth).
- Order thiamine 100 mg to prevent Wernicke's.
- Fluids can also be ordered with a multivitamin mixed in but verify that the patient will be receiving adequate thiamine.
- Pharmacologic options to add to the intravenous hydration include metoclopramide 5 to 10 mg every 8 hours, dimenhydrinate 50 mg every 4 to 6 hours, ondansetron 8 mg every 12 hours, and promethazine 12.5 to 25 mg every 4 to 6 hours.

- Refractory HG that is unresponsive to intravenous fluids and the previously mentioned medications may require chlorpromazine 25 to 50 mg every 4 to 6 hours or methylprednisolone 16 mg every 8 hours for 3 days.
- A patient with refractory HG may need enteral feeding.

> **CLINICAL PEARL:** HG may be present in patients with molar pregnancies, so be sure to check an ultrasound.

REFERENCE

1. American College of Obstetricians and Gynecologists. Practice bulletin no. 189. Nausea and vomiting of pregnancy. https://www.acog.org/Clinical%20Guidance%20and%20Publications/Practice%20Bulletins/Committee%20on%20Practice%20Bulletins%20Obstetrics/Nausea%20and%20Vomiting%20of%20Pregnancy.aspx. Published January 2018.

PLACENTAL ABRUPTION

Overview and Presentation

- Placental abruption is a common cause of third-trimester bleeding and can cause significant morbidity and mortality.[1,2]
- Patients with a placental abruption may present with vaginal bleeding, pain, and evidence of fetal distress on external fetal monitoring.
- The absence of vaginal bleeding does not rule out an abruption as the hemorrhage can remain intrauterine.
- Abdominal and pelvic pain can be abrupt in onset with subsequent abnormal uterine contractions.
- Maternal hypertension is the leading cause of placental abruption.
- An abruption can also be seen in patients with acute trauma, such as a motor vehicle accident, assault, or a fall.
- Tobacco use and cocaine use are strongly associated with risk of placental abruption.
- Placental abruption is associated with disseminated intravascular coagulopathy (DIC).

Diagnostic Evaluation

- A patient with late second- or third-trimester bleeding accompanied by abdominal or pelvic pain should have prompt assessment of vital signs and external fetal heart rate monitoring.

Management

- The management of an abruption requires a rapid response.
- Place large-bore intravenous access and begin infusing a crystalloid.

- Monitoring of blood pressure, heart rate, and blood loss is essential.
- Ensure continuous fetal heart rate monitoring.
- A Foley catheter will help quantify urine output.
- Laboratory studies include a CBC, type and cross, fibrinogen concentration, aPTT, and prothrombin time (PT).
- Evaluation of renal function and liver function can be helpful, particularly with severe bleeding or for preexisting preeclampsia or HELLP (hemolysis, elevated liver enzymes, low platelet count) syndrome.
- If illicit drug ingestion is suspected, a toxicology screen is also warranted.
- Transfusion of blood products depends on the clinical scenario, including severity of blood loss and possibility of developing DIC.
- A baseline hematocrit, platelets, and fibrinogen can be used to monitor progress with blood product transfusion.
- If fetal death has occurred, vaginal delivery is the preferred method of delivery. If the fetus is still alive, cesarean delivery will be performed.
- A vertical incision is usually the incision of choice as it is associated with less blood loss and is preferred for preterm pregnancies.

REFERENCES

1. Gaufberg SV. Emergent management of abruptio placentae. In: Lo BM, ed. *Medscape*. https://emedicine.medscape.com/article/795514-overview. Updated December 29, 2015.
2. Deering SH. Abruptio placentae treatment and management. In: Smith CV, ed. *Medscape*. https://emedicine.medscape.com/article/252810-treatment#d10 . Updated November 30, 2018.

POSTPARTUM HEMORRHAGE

Overview and Presentation

- Postpartum hemorrhage (PPH) is the leading cause of morbidity and mortality among pregnant patients worldwide.[1]
- The most common causes of primary PPH include uterine atony, lacerations, placenta accrete, retained placenta, coagulopathy, and uterine inversion.
- PPH has historically been defined as the loss of blood exceeding 500 mL in a vaginal delivery or 1,000 mL in a cesarean delivery, but ACOG recently redefined PPH as a cumulative blood loss of 1,000 mL or greater, or blood loss with evidence of hypovolemia that occurs within 24 hours after the intrapartum and/or postpartum period independent of mode of delivery.

Diagnostic Evaluation

- Careful examination of the patient to determine the source of bleeding is essential.

- Although abnormal uterine tone is the leading cause of postpartum hemorrhage, lacerations, retained placental tissue, and hematomas can also cause significant bleeding.

Management

- As soon as a PPH is suspected, the rapid response team should be notified.
- Uterine massage should continue.
- If not already in place, two large-bore intravenous catheters should be inserted and high-flow oxygen (10 to 15 L/min via face mask) should be administered.
- Isotonic crystalloids are the preferred fluids to help maintain urine output greater than 30 mL/hr.
- A balloon tamponade can be inserted if the patient is hemodynamically stable.
- Pharmacologic management includes use of oxytocin, methylergonovine, carboprost tromethamine, and tranexamic acid.
- Oxytocin dosing for intramuscular injection is 10 units with an expected response in 3 to 5 minutes.
- If oxytocin is given intravenously, use 40 units in 1 L of normal saline or lactated Ringer's but avoid a bolus injection of oxytocin.
- If bleeding continues, administer methylergonovine 200 mcg intramuscularly.
- The methylergonovine can be injected directly into the myometrium as well. Do not administer methylergonovine intravenously.
- A response should occur in 3 to 5 minutes, but if no improvement is seen, add carboprost tromethamine 250 mcg intramuscularly every 15 minutes for a maximum of eight doses.
- Carboprost should never be given intravenously and should be avoided in asthmatic patients.
- Tranexamic acid should be given within 3 hours of delivery and the dose is 1 g intravenously every 24 hours.
- Tranexamic acid is contraindicated in women with a history of a thromboembolic event.
- Initiation of tranexamic acid is associated with significant improvement in maternal and fetal survival.
- Blood products should be administered if hemodynamic status is not improving with fluids, usually starting with two units of packed red blood cells (RBCs) with plasma and platelets.
- Most institutions use a 1:1:1 ratio of RBCs: fresh frozen plasma (FFP): platelets.
- If DIC is suspected, cryoprecipitate should be administered.
- Surgical options include arterial embolization, laparotomy, and hysterectomy.
- The surgical decisions will depend on the hemodynamic status of the patient.

> **CLINICAL PEARL:** It is essential to monitor bleeding during and after delivery. A postpartum hemorrhage can occur within seconds and prompt recognition and intervention can mean the difference between life and death.

REFERENCE

1. American College of Obstetricians and Gynecologists. Practice bulletin no. 183. Postpartum hemorrhage. https://www.acog.org/Clinical-Guidance-and-Publications/Practice-Bulletins/Committee-on-Practice-Bulletins-Obstetrics/Postpartum-Hemorrhage. Published October 2017.

RETAINED PLACENTAL TISSUE

Overview and Presentation

- A placenta is not considered to be retained until 30 minutes after delivery.[1,2]
- A retained placenta may occur due to uterine atony or abnormalities of the placental decidua.
- Placenta accreta, history of retained placenta, preterm delivery, grand multiparity, and prior dilation and curettage are risk factors for the development of retained placenta.
- Retained placenta or retained placental tissue can occur when a patient has an abrupt hemorrhage despite an undelivered placenta. In fact, retained placenta is the second most common cause of postpartum hemorrhage, second only to uterine atony.
- A partial placental separation might have occurred, meaning that a portion of the placenta adheres to the uterus.
- Inspection of the delivered placenta may reveal missing membranes, placental fragments, or cotyledon.

Diagnostic Evaluation

- Ultrasound evaluation may be required when a patient presents postpartum with persistent heavy vaginal bleeding.

Management

- Manual removal can be attempted.
- A sterile glove should be placed over the existing glove on your dominant hand.

- A sterile towel is used to carefully sweep the uterus and remove the retained tissue.
- Refractory retained tissue may need surgical intervention.
- Retained tissue can cause hemorrhage and infection, so even after uncomplicated vaginal deliveries, the uterus is swept to ensure all clots and tissue have been removed.
- The World Health Organization recommends that if the placenta is not spontaneously expelled and hemorrhage is occurring, oxytocin 10 IU can be used.
- There is no role for the use of any uterotonic in retained placenta without hemorrhage.

> **CLINICAL PEARL:** Familiarize yourself with the normal appearance of the human placenta, both the maternal and fetal sides. When assisting in a delivery, ask to examine the placenta. Once you feel comfortable identifying a normal-appearing placenta, it will be much easier to identify abnormalities, such as missing pieces.

REFERENCES

1. Avery DM. Obstetric emergencies. *Am J Clin Med.* 2009;6(2):42–47. https://www.aapsus.org/wp-content/uploads/Obstetric-Emergencies.pdf
2. World Health Organization. *WHO Guidelines for the Management of Postpartum Hemorrhage and Retained Placenta.* Geneva, Switzerland: Author; 2009. http://apps.who.int/iris/bitstream/handle/10665/44171/9789241598514_eng.pdf; jsessionid=F0B07AA0B1C4AC486C3022143976D578?sequence=1

RUPTURED ECTOPIC PREGNANCY

Overview and Presentation

- All patients of reproductive age who present with a history of missed menses and pelvic pain should be considered to have an ectopic pregnancy until proven otherwise.[1]
- A ruptured ectopic pregnancy is more likely to occur in pregnancies that have implanted in the isthmus. Ampullary pregnancies tend to rupture later than isthmic pregnancies.
- A patient with missed menses, irregular vaginal bleeding, pelvic pain, syncope, abdominal pain, and/or dizziness should be managed as a ruptured ectopic pregnancy until proven otherwise.
- Ruptured ectopic pregnancies are associated with high mortality, particularly if diagnosis is delayed or missed.

Diagnostic Evaluation

- Physical examination of patients with a ruptured ectopic pregnancy can reveal pelvic tenderness, an adnexal mass, and evidence of hemodynamic compromise.
- A transvaginal ultrasound will often show an adnexal mass and/or fluid in the pouch of Douglas.
- The serum qualitative beta-human chorionic gonadotropin (beta-HCG) will be greater than 5 mIu/mL.

Management

- Immediately order a hemoglobin, hematocrit, type and cross, and place large-bore intravenous access for fluid support.
- Laparotomy is performed when patients are hemodynamically unstable or if visualization during laparoscopy was difficult.
- Patients with a ruptured ectopic pregnancy must be managed emergently and surgically.

> **CLINICAL PEARL:** A woman of reproductive age who presents with an acute abdomen should be ruled out for a ruptured ectopic pregnancy.

REFERENCE

1. Practice Bulletin No. 193. Tubal ectopic pregnancy. https://www.acog.org/Clinical-Guidance-and-Publications/Practice-Bulletins/Committee-on-Practice-Bulletins-Gynecology/Tubal-Ectopic-Pregnancy. Published March 2018.

SEXUAL ASSAULT

Overview and Presentation[1,2]

- *Rape* is defined as forceful anal or vaginal penetration with a penis or other object.[1,2]
  - Physical force does not need to be present as the Federal Bureau of Investigation's (FBI) definition includes sex with a person who is intoxicated and/or mentally and physically unable to provide consent.
- Most EDs employ a sexual assault nurse examiner or sexual assault forensic examiner to provide the evaluation and physical examination on a victim.
- If a victim presents to an outpatient office or other clinic, it is important to ensure that proper steps are followed in the collection of evidence because any improper technique can significantly alter the ability to prosecute the perpetrator.

- If a victim calls the office seeking advice, she must be instructed not to douche, bathe, or shower; change clothes; trim or clean her fingernails; eat/drink; urinate or defecate; or smoke.
- When a patient presents with sexual assault/rape, you must recognize early signs of life-threatening trauma such as hemorrhagic shock or head trauma.
- Once the patient has been deemed stable, provide a safe space for the patient, away from other patients and visitors.
- When documenting the history, try to use the patient's own words in quotation marks as much as possible.
- Obtain informed consent for the physical examination. The patient must be told that photographs may be taken but only if she provides consent.

Diagnostic Evaluation[1,2]

- When performing the physical examination, include the whole body.
- Do not only perform a pelvic examination. Remember, the body is the crime scene.
- Be prepared to document any abnormalities, such as bruises, lacerations, of other evidence of trauma.
- Samples are taken from under the fingernails, the vagina, oral or rectal cavity, pubic hair, dried blood, and any other foreign objects on the patient, such as hair.
- If anal penetration has occurred, you may need to perform proctoscopy.
- Note whether the hymen is intact and whether any other vulvovaginal or perineal trauma is present.
- Collect samples as needed.
- It is advised to test the patient for other sexually transmitted infections (STIs) with serology, such as rapid plasma reagin (RPR), HIV (rapid HIV testing is preferred), and hepatitis B and C.
- Also check the patient's blood type for comparison with the perpetrator.
- A pregnancy test can be ordered to make sure the patient is not already pregnant.

Management[1,2]

- Although few sexual assaults result in an STI, it is still advised to treat prophylactically for gonorrhea, chlamydia, and syphilis.
- Postexposure prophylaxis for HIV should be offered.
- You can also offer hepatitis B immunization if the patient is unaware of her status, but let the patient know that she will need a follow-up immunization in about 1 month.
- Emergency contraception should be offered.
  - The Food and Drug Administration (FDA) has approved levonorgestrel 0.75 mg, two oral tablets 12 hours apart, or levonorgestrel 1.5 mg as a single oral dose. A follow-up pregnancy test in 2 weeks is recommended.

- Report the assault to the appropriate authorities and allow the patient to be questioned if she consents and wants to report the assault.
- Child victims must be reported to the appropriate child protection agency.
- Sexual assault counseling should be initiated before the patient leaves the ED or the clinic.
- Make sure the patient has a safe place to go upon discharge and provide the patient with a follow-up appointment.

> **CLINICAL PEARL:** It is important to know your jurisdiction's time limit for collection of evidence as some have a 72-hour cutoff and others allow 1 week.

REFERENCES

1. American College of Obstetricians and Gynecologists. Committee opinion no. 777. Sexual assault. https://www.acog.org/Clinical-Guidance-and-Publications/Committee-Opinions/Committee-on-Health-Care-for-Underserved-Women/Sexual-Assault. Published March 26, 2019.
2. Marshall B, Marshall K. Obstetric and gynecologic emergencies and sexual assault. In: Belval B, Brown RY, eds. *Current Diagnosis and Treatment: Emergency Medicine.* 8th ed. New York, NY: McGraw-Hill Education; 2017:668–690.

THROMBOEMBOLISM

Overview and Presentation

- Pregnancy is a pro-thrombotic state.
- The physiological changes of pregnancy can mimic the signs and symptoms of pulmonary embolism (PE), so heightened clinical awareness of PE is imperative.
- Virchow's triad (venous stasis, hypercoagulability, and vascular injury) occurs physiologically during pregnancy and delivery, and risk for thromboembolic events continue through about 8 weeks' postpartum.
- About 80% of thromboembolic events are deep vein thrombosis (DVT) and about 20% are pulmonary emboli.[1]
- Most patients who present with an initial thromboembolic event in pregnancy do not have a documented coagulopathy.
- Risk factors include advanced maternal age, increased body mass index (BMI), multiparity, multiple gestation, tobacco use, autoimmune disorders, and hyperemesis gravidarum.[2]
- Thrombophilias, such as factor V Leiden, also increase a woman's risk for a thromboembolic event.
- Homan's sign has poor predictive value for a DVT.

Diagnostic Evaluation

- Any gravid woman who presents with unilateral calf pain or swelling should be ruled out for a DVT with a lower extremity compression duplex ultrasound.
- D-dimer measurement is not recommended.
- Initial diagnostic imaging for PE can include a chest radiograph to rule out pneumonia or effusions, but definitive diagnostic imaging with CT pulmonary angiography is considered the gold standard for PE.[2]
- Bilateral lower extremity compression duplex ultrasound should also be considered.

Management

- The initial treatment of thromboembolic events in pregnancy consists of low-molecular-weight heparin, such as enoxaparin 1 mg/kg every 12 hours. The recommended dose is 10,000 units subcutaneously every 12 hours, titrated to the target aPTT of 1.5 to 2.5, 6 hours after the injection. Low-molecular-weight and unfractionated heparins do not cross the placenta.[1]
- If heparin-induced thrombocytopenia occurs, fondaparinux is the preferred alternative.[1]
- Women can be converted to unfractionated heparin during the last 4 weeks of pregnancy.[1]
- In patients who are scheduled for a cesarean, cessation of anticoagulation typically begins 24 hours prior to the procedure.
- Pneumatic compression devices should be used as well.
- When women are deemed high risk (i.e., factor V Leiden), they can be given intravenous unfractionated heparin during labor.
- Reversal of anticoagulation with heparin is accomplished with protamine sulfate.
- Another option for high-risk women is to reduce the dose of anticoagulant to a prophylactic range.[1]
- Postpartum treatment with anticoagulants should begin within 4 to 6 hours after vaginal delivery and 6 to 12 hours post cesarean. Postpartum anticoagulation should continue for 4 to 6 weeks.[1]

> **CLINICAL PEARL:** In patients who are diagnosed with a thromboembolic event during pregnancy, it is reasonable to screen for factor V Leiden, antiphospholipid antibodies, and protein C and S deficiencies.

REFERENCES

1. American College of Obstetricians and Gynecologists. Practice Bulletin No. 196. Thromboembolism in pregnant. https://www.acog.org/Clinical-Guidance-and-Publications/Practice-Bulletins/Committee-on-Practice-Bulletins-Obstetrics/Thromboembolism-in-Pregnancy. Published June 25, 2018.
2. Simcox LE, Ormesher L, Tower C, Greer IA. Pulmonary thromboembolism in pregnancy: diagnosis and management. *Breathe*. 2015;11(4):282–289. doi:10.1183/20734735.008815

TUBO-OVARIAN ABSCESS

Overview and Presentation

- A tubo-ovarian abscess (TOA) is a complex infectious mass of the adnexa that forms as a sequela of pelvic inflammatory disease.[1]
- Classically, a TOA manifests with an adnexal mass, fever, elevated white blood cell count, lower abdominal–pelvic pain, and/or vaginal discharge; however, presentations of this disease can be highly variable.
- Should the abscess rupture, life-threatening sepsis can occur.

Diagnostic Evaluation

- CBC with differential may show leukocytosis and a left shift.
- Physical examination must include a pelvic examination to check for the presence of cervicitis, cervical motion tenderness, and adnexal tenderness or a mass.
- A beta-HCG must be performed to rule out pregnancy.
- Pelvic ultrasonography will reveal a complex cystic mass.

Management

- Surgical intervention is undertaken when rupture is suspected or if the patient is not responding to antibiotics.
- The Centers for Disease Control and Prevention (CDC) recommends the following antibiotic regimen.
  ○ Cefoxitin 2 g intravenously every 6 hours or cefotetan 2 g intravenously every 12 hours plus doxycycline 100 mg every 12 hours, either intravenously or orally and anaerobic coverage with clindamycin or metronidazole.
  ○ An alternative regimen is clindamycin 900 mg intravenously every 8 hours plus gentamicin 2 mg/kg as a loading dose, followed by 1.5 mg/kg every 8 hours.
  ○ Antibiotics should be continued until the fever normalizes, the white blood cell count returns to normal, pain resolves, and a decrease in the size of the abscess is confirmed.

- A ruptured TOA is a surgical emergency.
- Patients with a ruptured abscess will have evidence of peritonitis.
- Sepsis can occur rapidly and subsequent mortality is high in these patients.

Reference

1. Centers for Disease Control and Prevention. 2015 sexually transmitted diseases treatment guidelines. Pelvic inflammatory disease (PID). https://www.cdc.gov/std/tg2015/pid.htm

7

Common Procedures in Gynecology

BARTHOLIN CYST OR ABSCESS INCISION AND DRAINAGE

Indication

Patients with a Bartholin gland cyst or abscess must undergo incision and drainage followed by insertion of a Word catheter or, if a Word catheter is unavailable, gauze packing. Recurrent cysts or abscesses should undergo biopsy and marsupialization.

Equipment

- Absorbent pads
- Sterile gloves
- Sterile procedure drapes
- Sterile betadine or other topical skin cleanser
- Topical lidocaine gel
- Lidocaine 1% without epinephrine
- Normal saline
- 3-mL syringe and 25- or 27-gauge needle for anesthesia injection
- 5-mL syringe filled with normal saline for Word catheter balloon inflation
- 10-mL syringe filled with sterile water for irrigation of wound after incision and drainage
- No. 11 scalpel
- Several 4 × 4 gauze pads
- Sterile iodiform gauze for packing (if a Word catheter is not available)
- Hemostat for breaking up loculations

- Culture swab for abscesses
- Word catheter

Procedure[1]

1. Obtain written informed consent after discussing the risks, benefits, and alternatives of the procedure to the patient.
2. Place the patient in the lithotomy position and ensure adequate draping.
3. Place absorbent pad under the patient's buttocks.
4. Cleanse the area with betadine or other skin cleanser.
5. Topical and local anesthesia can be applied prior to the incision.
   - If using injectable anesthesia, it is sometimes helpful to apply lidocaine 2% gel or benzocaine 20% gel to the vulva prior to injection.
   - Inject the anesthetic into the vulva below the level of the cyst or abscess.
   - Do not inject directly into the cyst or abscess.
6. Follow appropriate sterile procedures.
7. Using a No. 11 blade, incise the cyst or abscess on the inner labial surface.
8. The incision should be at least 0.5 cm to allow for insertion of a Word catheter or gauze.
9. Using a hemostat or your fingers, express all fluid from the mass.
10. If an abscess is present, use a culture swab to collect fluid but be careful to avoid contamination by touching the patient's external genitalia.
11. Copiously irrigate the wound.
12. If a Word catheter is available, insert the catheter directly into the wound and inflate the balloon with 4 mL of normal saline.
13. If a Word catheter is not available, pack the wound with sterile gauze.
14. Insert the end of the catheter into the vagina.
15. The catheter should be left in place for several weeks.
16. Sitz baths are commonly recommended for the first few days after the procedure.
17. If gauze packing is used, it should be removed within 48 hours.
18. Patients should abstain from sexual intercourse for the duration of placement of the Word catheter.

> **CLINICAL PEARL:** Marsupialization is an outpatient surgical procedure that involves surgical resection of the Bartholin gland cyst. It sometimes can be performed in the office but should not be performed if an abscess is present.

REFERENCE

1. Shlamovitz GZ. Bartholin abscess drainage. In: Isaacs C, ed. *Medscape.* https://emedicine.medscape.com/article/80260-overview#a8. Updated January 8, 2019.

Colposcopy

Indication

A colposcope is a large binocular magnifying instrument used to evaluate the vulva, vagina, perineum, anus, and cervix in women with various issues, including an abnormal Pap test or a suspicious lesion. The procedure allows for direct visualization of abnormal tissue followed by biopsy for confirmatory diagnosis. Colposcopy can be performed during pregnancy, but cervical and endocervical biopsies should not be performed. All colposcopic evaluations require written informed consent prior to the procedure, and no anesthesia is necessary, but some providers use a topical benzocaine application to the vulva or the cervix prior to performing a biopsy.

Equipment

- Colposcope
- Speculum
- Monsel's solution
- Acetic acid
- Lugol's iodine solution
- Large cotton-tip applicators (at least six) or cotton balls that will be attached to ring forceps
- Endocervical speculum (if you need to augment the transformation zone)
- Endocervical curette
- Cervical punch biopsy forceps
- Formalin jars (at least three)

Procedure (for Cervical Biopsy)

1. Make sure the patient has had a negative pregnancy test prior to the procedure.
2. Make sure written consent has been obtained.
3. Ensure all equipment is ready and within easy reach.
4. Place the patient in the lithotomy position and ensure adequate draping.
5. Insert the speculum with posterior (downward) pressure to avoid the clitoris.
6. Visualize the cervix and lock the speculum.
7. Insert large cotton-tip applicators or cotton balls attached to ring forceps that have been soaked in 3% to 5% acetic acid solution (vinegar) to coat the cervix. Some providers use iodine and potassium iodide (Lugol's solution) to visualize the cervix. Lugol's is better to evaluate vaginal lesions.
8. After the cotton balls or cotton-tip applicators are removed, the colposcope is placed at the foot of the bed, about 12″ from the introitus, and the cervix is visualized through the lens. Just as when you look through a standard microscope, you will likely have to adjust the settings for your

vision and distance from the site. There are important steps to follow when performing colposcopy.

9. Identify the transformation zone. This is the metaplastic squamous epithelium that lies between the original squamocolumnar junction and the active squamocolumnar junction. If the transformation zone cannot be visualized, use the endocervical speculum. If you still cannot identify the transformation zone, the colposcopy is considered unsatisfactory.

10. Scan the entire surface of the cervix, looking for abnormalities. Intraepithelial lesions can be graded based on specific findings. Mosacisim and punctation reflect abnormal vascularity; larger and more coarse findings generally correlate with higher grade lesions. Vacularity that appears atypical, such as having a comma or corkscrew shape, is associated with invasive disease. Abnormal cells will become acetopositive, meaning they will turn a whitish color.

11. A green filter is available on colposcopes. Use of the green filter allows for better visualization of vascularity. Blood vessels will appear black when visualized with the colposcope.

12. Biopsies of the cervix are taken with cervical biopsy forceps. Kevorkian–Younge and Tischler are common forceps. The size of the biopsy will be 3 to 5 mm. Each biopsy sample will be placed in a separate formalin jar with the appropriate location of site of biopsy labeled.

13. After all punch biopsies are obtained, an endocervical sample is obtained, usually with a special curette. However, an endocervical brush can be used, but it is important to insert into the endocervical canal, much deeper than when taking a Pap sample.

14. Apply Monsel's solution to all biopsy sites for hemostasis. Monsel's solution is a mustardy-yellow, pasty mixture of ferric sulfate, ferrous sulfate, and sterile water. Monsel's solution is applied to the biopsy sites using large cotton-tipped applicators. Apply the solution to the cervix and use a bit of pressure to help stop bleeding. There is no need to "pack" the vagina after the procedure. The combination of blood and Monsel's creates a coffee-ground appearance. It is important to let the patient know that she will see some of this after the procedure. Give the patient a pantiliner before she gets dressed.

15. Document abnormal findings by artificially dividing the cervix as if the cervix was a clock face. Small punch biopsies are obtained from the areas of concern and labeled with the anatomic area of the cervix. For example, biopsy no. 1 from 9:00, biopsy no. 2 from 6:00. Each biopsy specimen will be sent to pathology in a separate formalin jar labeled with the corresponding anatomic site. This is labeled *endocervical curette*. Again, biopsy and endometrial sampling should not be performed in pregnancy.

16. Advise the patient not to use tampons, to douche, or have sexual intercourse for 1 week after the procedure, and to report any unusual discharge.

17. Allow the patient a few minutes to rest. It may be helpful to have her lay on her side prior to getting up.
18. Let the patient know results should be back within 1 week.

CLINICAL PEARL: Becoming a skilled colposcopist takes time and mentoring. Consider attending a continuing-education seminar on introductory and advanced colposcopy once you have passed your boards.

ENDOMETRIAL BIOPSY

Indication

Endometrial biopsies (EMBs) are indicated when there is a suspicion for endometrial hyperplasia or cancer, irregular menstrual bleeding, prolonged amenorrhea, and even in the evaluation of a patient with infertility. EMB is contraindicated in patients who are pregnant, have cervical cancer, or who have pelvic inflammatory disease or a vaginal or cervical infection. Written informed consent must be obtained prior to the procedure. It is advisable to have the patient take a nonsteroidal anti-inflammatory drug (NSAID) 1 hour prior to the procedure, unless there are contraindications to NSAID use. An EMB can be performed in the office without any anesthesia, but some providers will use topical benzocaine spray. Benzocaine spray or gel can be used to help with the discomfort of tenaculum placement. EMB is considered a sterile procedure so it is important to pay close attention to technique so as not to contaminate the sterile field.[1]

Equipment
- Speculum
- Large cotton-tip applicators (at least two) or cotton balls that will be attached to ring forceps, soaked in povidone-iodine solution or chlorhexidine)
- Tenaculum
- Povidone-iodine solution
- Uterine sound
- Endometrial pipelle
- Formalin jar
- Benzocaine spray or gel (provider dependent)

Procedure
1. Obtain informed consent from the patient.
2. If the patient is of reproductive age, make sure a recent pregnancy test is negative.

3. Place the patient in the lithotomy position and ensure adequate draping.

4. Insert the speculum with posterior (downward) pressure to avoid the clitoris.

5. Visualize the cervix and lock the speculum.

6. Cleanse the cervix with the povidone-iodine solution (unless the patient is allergic in which case you can use chlorhexidine).

7. A tenaculum can be placed along the anterior lip of the cervix for stabilization.

8. Measure the uterine cavity with a uterine sound with extreme care not to contaminate the sound or perforate the uterus. Most uterine depths will be 6 to 8 cm, from the external cervical os to the fundus. Sometimes the internal os creates difficult passage of the sound. A small Pratt dilator can be used to aid in the passage of the sound. In postmenopausal patients, the internal os can be quite rigid. Some providers will place a seaweed osmotic laminaria in the cervix the morning of the procedure. The patient can return in the afternoon for the EMB.

9. Now that you know the measure of the uterine depth, insert the pipelle with care not to exceed the depth of the uterus.

10. A pipelle is a flexible cannula with suction capabilities that is inserted into the uterine cavity to obtain endometrial tissue. Withdrawing the piston from the catheter creates suction. Withdraw the internal piston and move the pipelle up and down the uterine cavity without completely withdrawing the pipelle and rotate the pipelle 360 degrees during movement. A minimum of four passes should be made.

11. Once the catheter is filled with endometrial tissue, withdraw the catheter and place the tissue in a properly labeled formalin jar by reinserting the piston and forcing the tissue out. Some providers will perform a second uterine sampling. If this is performed, it is imperative to ensure the catheter is not contaminated.

12. After adequate sampling has been obtained, remove the tenaculum and then the speculum. Pull out the end of the table and have the patient remove her legs from the stirrups. Allow the patient a few minutes to rest. It may be helpful to have her lay on her side prior to getting up.

CLINICAL PEARL: Use of intravaginal misoprostol 25 mcg the night before the procedure can help soften the cervix prior to the procedure.

REFERENCE

1. Gordon P. Endometrial biopsy. Videos in clinical medicine. *N Engl J Med.* 2009;361:e61. doi:10.1056/NEJMvcm0803922

Intrauterine System Removal

Indication

Women present for intrauterine system (IUS) removals for various reasons. Some women may report that their partner can feel the strings and thus they want it removed. Others will report side effects that they feel they cannot endure. Some will have one removed when the life span of the IUS is expiring and may want another reinserted at the same visit. And others will want it removed when they are ready to attempt conception. Appropriate patient education is necessary for all patients presenting with the desire to have their IUS removed.

Equipment

- Ring forceps
- Alligator forceps
- Cytobrush (if the strings cannot readily be visualized)
- Intrauterine device (IUD) hook (if strings cannot readily be visualized)
- Sterile container for IUS culture if chronic cervicitis or pelvic inflammatory disease (PID) is suspected

Procedure

1. Obtain informed consent for IUS removal.
2. Discuss with the patient what type of contraception she would like to use once the IUS has been removed.
3. Place the patient in the lithotomy position and ensure adequate draping.
4. Note that removal of an IUS does not require sterile technique.
5. Insert the speculum using posterior (downward) pressure and visualize the cervix.
6. Lock the speculum in place.
7. Visualize the strings at the cervical os.
   a. Sometimes you will need to insert a cytobrush into the endocervical canal to try and locate the strings.
   b. If you still cannot visualize the strings, try using an IUD hook.
   c. If you still cannot visualize the strings, you may need an ultrasound to locate the device as malpositioning can occur.
8. Use a ring forceps or alligator forceps to grasp the strings.
9. It is helpful to have the patient give a strong cough; while she coughs, pull firmly on the strings.
10. You may consider sending the IUS to the lab for culture if the patient appears to have PID or chronic cervicitis.
11. Provide patient education on contraceptive options, if the patient does not wish to conceive.

> **CLINICAL PEARL:** Ask the patient whether she wants to see the removed IUS before discarding it.

PAP TEST/HUMAN PAPILLOMAVIRUS SCREENING

Indication

A Papanicolaou test, formerly called a *Pap smear*, is a fundamental task in OB/GYN. Pap tests screen for cervical dysplasia and cancer but are not used solely for diagnosing dysplasia or cancer. Under certain circumstances, abnormal Pap results mean that the patient must have a colposcopy with or without biopsy, depending on what the colposcopist visualizes and whether the patient is pregnant. The human papilloma virus (HPV) is responsible for almost all abnormalities of the cervix. In the past, women underwent Pap testing annually, but retrospective studies showed that over 90% of otherwise healthy young women would clear an HPV infection on their own, without any medical intervention. In addition, the presence or absence of high-risk HPV (most common are 16 and 18, but there are others) is perhaps more informative than the cytologic report. Thus, the ASCCP (formerly called the *American Society for Colposcopy and Cervical Pathology*) has published detailed algorithms regarding the screening and management of abnormal Pap tests (https://www.asccp.org/Guidelines).

Equipment

- Speculum
- Light source
- Small amount of lubricant
- Cytology collection system (a liquid-based system is the most commonly used; cytobrush, spatula, or broom). Commercially prepared Pap test kits are utilized extensively in offices and clinics, so if unsure about what to use, ask a nurse or medical assistant.

Procedure

1. Before performing a Pap test or any other pelvic examination, make sure all equipment is readily available within reaching distance.
2. Place the patient in the lithotomy position and ensure adequate draping.
3. Insert the speculum using posterior (downward) pressure to avoid hitting the clitoris.

4. After you insert the speculum, locate the cervix. Sometimes the cervix will be facing posteriorly or anteriorly and you will have to maneuver the speculum. It can be helpful to have the patient place her hands under her buttocks to lift the pelvis if she is obese and you are having a difficult time with visualization.

5. Once you have the cervix in view, lock the speculum.

6. Always make note of what you see before and after the Pap test. For example, if there are visible lesions or growths, such as Nebothian cysts or endocervical polyps, make sure you document those findings in the note. If there is significant bleeding with the Pap test, this must be documented because friability can be associated with dysplasia, cancer, and cervicitis.

7. When performing the actual Pap test, make sure you rotate the device (spatula, brush, and/or broom) at least 360 degrees around the cervical os. You want to make sure you apply enough pressure to obtain cells from the transformation zone and endocervix, but not enough that you go so deeply as to inadvertently perform an endometrial biopsy.

8. Remove the speculum by first unlocking it and then slowly letting it close on itself, again using posterior (downward) pressure to avoid the clitoris.

9. An example of what you may write about a patient with a normal exam:

   a. Cervix was adequately visualized and had no Nabothian cysts, polyps, or other lesions. There was no discharge from the os. The broom was used for collection of cells and adequately rotated at least 360 degrees. No bleeding after the Pap test and the patient tolerated the procedure well.

   b. Then, after you perform a bimanual exam, the cervical portion of the exam would read: The cervix was long and closed with no cervical motion tenderness on bimanual exam.

> **CLINICAL PEARL:** The Pap test (and any pelvic examination) can be distressing for many women. Be sure to provide emotional support as necessary and be as quick, but thorough, as possible. It is advisable to have a chaperone in the room as well.

VULVAR BIOPSY

Indication

Women with chronic vulvar pruritus or the presence of a suspicious lesion on the vulva should undergo vulvar biopsy. Common causes of chronic pruritus include lichen sclerosis and lichen simplex chronicus; vulvar neoplasia; squamous cell carcinoma; and Paget disease.[1]

Equipment

- Colposcope (if the lesion is not readily visible)
- Lugol's solution if using colposcopy
- Small needle (27-G or 30-G)
- Small syringe filled with 1% to 2 % local anesthetic without epinephrine
- A No. 11 or No. 15 blade for raised lesions
- Small sterile forceps
- Sterile iris scissors
- Punch biopsy (4 or 5 mm) for flat or slightly raised lesions
- Povidone-iodine or chlorhexidine
- Monsel's solution or silver nitrate stick for hemostasis
- Formalin jar(s)

Procedure

1. Obtain informed consent from the patient.
2. Place the patient in the lithotomy position and ensure adequate draping.
3. Cleanse the vulva or area that you will biopsy with chlorhexidine or iodine.
4. If using a colposcope, place Lugol's solution on the vulva and visualize the vulva through the colposcope.
5. Use a small needle (such as a 27-G or 30-G) to inject 1% to 2% of local anesthetic without epinephrine into the area of interest.
6. If the lesion is raised or pedunculated, you can use a sterile blade (such as a No. 11 or No. 15) or sterile scissors to remove the lesion. If the lesion is not amenable to a scalpel or scissors, such as flat or slightly raised lesions, use a standard punch biopsy.
7. If performing a punch biopsy, place the punch biopsy on the skin, apply some pressure to allow for penetration through the epithelium, and rotate the punch biopsy clockwise and counterclockwise. Avoid making multiple rotations.
8. Use forceps to raise the specimen and sterile scissors or a scalpel to cut the base.
9. Regardless of technique, the sample will be placed in a specimen jar with appropriate fixative and sent to the pathologist.
10. As the vulva is quite vascular, there can be bleeding after the biopsy. Often, bleeding can be easily controlled with pressure, but you can use Monsel's solution or a silver nitrate stick. Be careful only to apply the hemostatic agent to the area that is bleeding and avoid surrounding tissue. Larger biopsies may require suture placement. A 4-0 monofilament or polygalactin suture is generally sufficient.
11. It is difficult to place bandages on the vulva, so provide the patient with a pantiliner to use.

12. Provide post procedure education:
    a. Advise the patient that she must keep the area clean and dry as possible.
    b. It usually takes 5 to 7 days for complete healing.
    c. Bathing is fine during this time, but the patient should not go in a hot tub until the wound is completely healed.
    d. If the biopsy required suturing, it is best to advise the patient to wait 24 hours to shower or bathe.
    e. The patient should report any unusual bleeding or discharge.
    f. Results should be back within 1 week.

> **CLINICAL PEARL:** Any suspicious vulvar lesion should be biopsied. If the lesion appears too large for an adequate punch biopsy, consider referral to dermatology or a gynecologic oncologist.

REFERENCE

1. American College of Obstetricians and Gynecologists. Practice bulletin no. 93. Diagnosis and management of vulvar skin disorders. https://www.acog.org/Clinical-Guidance-and-Publications/Practice-Bulletins/Committee-on-Practice-Bulletins-Gynecology/Diagnosis-and-Management-of-Vulvar-Skin-Disorders. Published May 2008. Reaffirmed 2019.

8

Common Procedures in Obstetrics

Cesarean Delivery

Indication

Cesarean deliveries can be scheduled or performed in an emergency situation. Primary cesareans usually occur due to labor dystocia, abnormal fetal heart rate patterns, malpresentation of the fetus (breech), multiple gestation, arrest of labor, and fetal macrosomia. Cesarean delivery will also be performed if the patient has an active outbreak of herpes simplex virus. The American College of Obstetricians and Gynecologists (ACOG) supports efforts to reduce unnecessary primary cesarean deliveries by clarifying the definition of arrest of labor. The surgical procedure of a cesarean involves several steps. Each surgeon will have his or her own particularities, but the general flow of the procedure is outlined as follows:[1,2]

Six centimeters of cervical dilation is the threshold for the active phase of labor. Arrest of labor during the first stage is defined by 6 cm or more of dilation, with rupture of membranes, and either 4 or more hours of adequate uterine contractions or 6 or more hours of inadequate contractions with no cervical change despite oxytocin. In addition, ACOG recommends the following:

Prolonged latent phase of labor, defined as more than 20 hours in a nullipara or more than 14 hours in a multipara, should not, on its own, be a requirement for cesarean delivery. Arrest of labor during the second stage should not be diagnosed until 2 or more hours of active pushing in multiparas or 3 or more hours of active pushing in nulliparas.

Equipment
- Mayo scissors (straight and curved)
- Hemostats (curved)

- Mayo Hager needle holder
- Heany needle holder
- Scalpel handle
- Scalpel blades
- Dissection forceps
- Tissue forceps
- Kelly forceps (straight and curved)
- Crile forceps
- Allis tissue forceps
- Backhaus towel forceps
- Retractors (Doyen and Kelly)
- Sponge forceps
- Cord clamps
- Suture material
- Laparotomy sponges

Procedure

1. Women who undergo nonemergent cesarean delivery will have been on nothing per os status (NPO) for at least 6 hours, have a Foley catheter in place, intravenous hydration, and cefazolin 1 to 2 g intravenously for prophylaxis.
2. Deep vein thrombosis prophylaxis with mechanical or pharmacologic interventions will be initiated.
3. Skin/abdominal incision: The most common incision is the Pfannenstiel.
   a. The incision will extend beyond the lateral aspects of the rectus muscles bilaterally and into the fascia.
   b. The fascia is then incised along the length of the initial incision.
   c. Using sharp and blunt dissection, the rectus muscles are separated from the fascia.
   d. Two curved hemostats are used to grasp the peritoneum and separated with a curved Metzenbaum scissors.
   e. The peritoneum is entered. At this point, the surgeon will be exceptionally careful not to injure the bladder or the bowel.
4. Bladder flap: Most surgeons will create a bladder flap at this point. The surgeon will dissect the bladder from the lower uterine segment, grasp the peritoneum, and make an incision with Metzenbaum scissors.
   a. A bladder blade is used to protect the bladder and to expose the lower uterine segment.
5. Uterine incision/hysterotomy: Incision choice is determined by the gestational age of the pregnancy, the placental location, fetal presentation, and how long the patient has been laboring. The most common uterine incision is a low transverse (also called a *Monroe–Kerr*).
   a. A low transverse incision is 1 to 2 cm above where the bladder would normally be located.

    b. The incision is only deep enough to allow visualization of fetal membranes or entry into the uterus.

    c. The surgeon will then use his or her index finger or bandage scissors to bluntly dissect the uterine incision with subsequent delivery of the fetus.

6. Once the fetus has been delivered, the umbilical cord is clamped and cut, and blood is retrieved from the umbilical cord for fetal blood typing.

    a. If blood gases are required, a segment of cord will be set aside.

7. The placenta is then delivered and inspected.

8. Oxytocin 20 units is administered into the intravenous line.

9. Uterine repair: The surgeon will allow for spontaneous expulsion of the placenta via uterine massage; some surgeons will manually remove the uterine fundus from the abdominal cavity for inspection, uterine massage, and manual removal of the placenta, if necessary.

    a. A dry laparotomy sponge is used to wipe the uterine cavity of membranes and any other debris.

    b. The surgeon will usually use a 0 or 2-0 polyglactin or chromic suture material in a one- or two-layer closure. ACOG recommends using a two-layer closure in women who desire to attempt vaginal birth after cesarean (VBAC) in subsequent pregnancies, but many surgeons will perform a one-layer closure.

    c. After checking for hemostasis and the integrity of the bladder, the uterus is then replaced.

    d. The peritoneum may be sutured. Most surgeons will not reapproximate and suture the rectus muscles.

    e. The fascia is closed using a running, nonlocking stitch but chromic sutures are generally not used for this layer.

    f. A subcutaneous incision greater than 2 cm may benefit from subcutaneous reapproximation and suturing. Staples or subcuticular sutures are then placed to complete closure.

10. Postoperatively, vital signs are obtained every 15 minutes for the first hour or 2 and urine output is measured hourly.

11. Intravenous fluids are usually continued throughout the first 24 hours but the patient can begin clear fluids within 12 hours if the operation was uncomplicated.

CLINICAL PEARL: Postoperative wound checks are important as wound dehiscence, particularly in obese women, is common, and it is important to check for bacterial colonization. Sometimes obese women with a large pannus will develop a secondary skin fungal infection as well. Patient education on good wound hygiene is critical.

REFERENCES

1. American College of Obstetricians and Gynecologists. Safe prevention of the primary cesarean delivery. Obstetric care consensus no. 1. https://www.acog .org/Clinical-Guidance-and-Publications/Obstetric-Care-Consensus-Series/Safe -Prevention-of-the-Primary-Cesarean-Delivery. Published March 2014. Reaffirmed 2019.
2. Saint Louis H. Cesarean delivery. In: Isaacs C, ed. *Medscape.* https:// emedicine.medscape.com/article/263424-overview. Updated December 14, 2018.

DELAYED CORD CLAMPING

Indication

In 2017, ACOG published a Committee Opinion regarding delayed umbilical cord clamping. According to ACOG, at least 30 to 60 seconds of delayed clamping in otherwise "vigorous" term and preterm infants should be performed. Delayed clamping results in increased hemoglobin in the newborn and improves overall iron stores during the first few months of a newborn's life. Delayed clamping does not increase the risk of postpartum hemorrhage. In preterm infants, the benefits of delayed cord clamping are numerous. These benefits include decreased risk of blood transfusion, improved red blood cell volume, and decreased risk of intraventricular hemorrhage and necrotizing enterocolitis. Delayed cord clamping should not be performed in certain situations such as maternal hemorrhage, placental abruption, or the need for newborn resuscitation. ACOG acknowledges that a small increase in jaundice that may necessitate phototherapy may occur. Adequate follow-up of infants regarding possible jaundice is required.[1]

Equipment

- Umbilical cord clamp

Procedure

1. After delivery, delay clamping for 30 to 60 seconds.
2. The infant can be placed on the maternal abdomen during the delay.

CLINICAL PEARL: Delayed clamping can be accomplished after a cesarean delivery but only in nonurgent or emergent situations.

REFERENCE

1. American College of Obstetricians and Gynecologists. Delayed umbilical cord clamping after birth. Committee opinion no. 684. https://www.acog.org/Clinical-Guidance-and-Publications/Committee-Opinions/Committee-on-Obstetric-Practice/Delayed-Umbilical-Cord-Clamping-After-Birth. Published January 2017. Reaffirmed 2018.

INDUCTION OF LABOR

Indication

Over 20% of pregnant women will undergo labor induction in the United States. ACOG supports efforts to reduce inappropriate labor inductions. In normal gestations before 39 weeks, and with an unfavorable cervix, there must be a strong medical reason to induce a patient. Induction of labor can be accomplished through several different interventions. The Bishop score will allow the provider an objective measurement as to the potential success or failure of the induction (see Bishop score). Bishop scores of less than 6 are associated with a two fold increase in risk of cesarean delivery. Nulliparous women should have a Bishop score higher than 8 and multiparous women should have a Bishop score greater than 6 prior to considering induction.[1-3]

Some fetal and maternal issues require earlier delivery and thus, induction would be medically appropriate. In pregnancies of 34 weeks' gestation or more, common reasons for medical induction include placenta previa, prior myomectomy, fetal growth restriction, multiple gestations, oligohydramnios, hypertensive disorders in pregnancy, and diabetes that is not well controlled. Please note that in twin gestations with complications, delivery may be indicated as early as 32w0d.

Induction of labor is contraindicated in the following settings:

- History of uterine rupture
- History of classical cesarean incision
- History of a transmural uterine incision for myomectomy
- Placenta previa or vasa previa
- Umbilical cord prolapse
- Current genital herpes infection
- Fetal malposition (transverse lie)

Equipment

- Transcervical Foley catheter or Cook balloon
- Prostaglandin E2 (PG2; dinoprostone)
- Prostaglandin E1 (PG1; misoprostol)
- Oxytocin infusion

- Tocodynamometer
- Amniotomy device (finger cot with a hook or a 10″ rod-shaped device with a hook)

Procedure

1. All inductions must be done in the labor and delivery unit where adequate nursing monitoring can be accomplished
2. Cervical ripening
   a. Transcervical Foley catheters or Cook balloons
   b. PG2 (dinoprostone)
      i. Available in a 2.5-mL syringe with 0.5 mg gel and a vaginal insert with 10 mg
      ii. Oxytocin administration is delayed for 6 to 12 hours after administration
   c. PG1 (misoprostol)
      i. Can be given sublingually, intravaginally, or orally.
      ii. Usual dose is 25 mcg.
      iii. Risk of uterine tachysystole at doses greater than 50 mcg; delay oxytocin administration for 4 hours.
   d. Combination of transcervical Foley and PG1.
3. Stripping of membranes
   a. Stripping the membranes causes increases in prostaglandin F2a and phospholipase A2.
   b. Stripping (or sweeping) of membranes is often done at the patient's prenatal visit using a sterile glove.
   c. The patient must be advised that she may experience vaginal spotting and pelvic cramping.
   d. Avoid stripping of membranes if the patient is positive for group B *Streptococcus* (GBS).
4. Oxytocin administration
   a. Administration of oxytocin requires careful monitoring of the cardiotocograph to identify uterine tachysystole and poor fetal response to contractions.
   b. Oxytocin should be diluted to an oxytocin concentration of 10 units/mL and administered by an infusion pump that allows for accurate control of the rate.
   c. There are two regimens used for oxytocin administration, a high dose and a low dose.
   d. The regimen chosen will depend on the clinical scenario, and each carries its own risks and advantages.
   e. A low-dose regimen may begin with 0.5 to 2 mU/min with an increase of 1 to 2 mU/min every 15 to 40 minutes.
   f. A high-dose regimen may begin at 6 mU/min with an increase of 3 to 6 mU/min every 15 to 40 minutes.

5. Amniotomy[2]
   a. Amniotomy is a procedure performed by an obstetrical provider to artificially rupture the amniotic sac. There are two instruments used for amniotomy; one is a 10″ rod-shaped device with a hook on the end, and the other is a finger cot with a hook on the end.
   b. Prior to performing amniotomy it is imperative to assess cervical dilation, fetal presentation, and fetal station. If the fetal caput is not adequately engaged, umbilical cord prolapse can occur. Indeed, this is the most common complication of amniotomy and if it occurs, will cause fetal distress due to cord compression, and emergency cesarean delivery is performed.

> **CLINICAL PEARL:** Nulliparous patients should have a modified Bishop score of at least 5 or a Bishop score of at least 8 in order to be considered for an induction. Scores less than these are associated with failed inductions.

REFERENCES

1. American College of Obstetricians and Gynecologists. Practice bulletin no. 107. Induction of labor. https://www.acog.org/Clinical-Guidance-and-Publications/Practice-Bulletins/Committee-on-Practice-Bulletins-Obstetrics/Induction-of-Labor. Published August 2009. Reaffirmed 2019.
2. Glowacki C, Whitten RA. Amniotomy. In: Gossman W, ed., *StatPearls*. Treaure Island, FL: StatsPearl; 2019. https://www.ncbi.nlm.nih.gov/books/NBK470167
3. Laughon SK, Zhang J, Troendle J, et al. Using a simplified Bishop score to predict vaginal delivery. *Obstet Gynecol*. 2011;117:805–811. doi:10.1097/AOG.0b013e3182114ad2

NONSTRESS TEST

Indication

There are various noninvasive methods to evaluate fetal health and the nonstress test (NST) is the most common. NSTs can be used after 28 weeks' gestation when the fetus' central nervous system is mature enough to respond to sympathetic and parasympathetic changes. For most indications, NST and biophysical profiles begin at 32 weeks. In some patients with severe anomalies, testing could be initiated at 26 weeks. There is little consensus regarding how often to perform NSTs, but they are usually done either every week or twice a week. Common indications for an NST include decreased fetal movement as reported by the mother and the presence of comorbid medical problems, such as hypertension, preeclampsia, diabetes, and autoimmune disorders. Some OB/GYN providers have women who are considered to be at advanced maternal age (>35 years) undergo routine NSTs starting at 32 weeks' gestation.[1]

Equipment
- Tocodynamometer

Procedure
1. This test is done in an outpatient setting, or in a separate NST room on the labor and delivery floor.
2. The patient is placed in the semi-Fowler position (seated, head elevated 30 degrees).
3. Two belts are placed around the gravid mother's uterus. One is to document fetal heart rate, and the other is to document the presence of uterine contractions.
4. The mother holds a device that she clicks whenever she feels the baby move. A notch is recorded on the paper strip, and the evaluator can assess the fetal heart rate's reaction to its own movement or a uterine contraction.
5. See Chapter 4, Diagnostic Testing for OB/GYN Conditions, for more information about NST interpretation.

CLINICAL PEARL: If the fetus appears to be in a sleep cycle, provide the patient with ice water or fruit juice if the patient is not diabetic.

REFERENCE

1. American College of Obstetricians and Gynecologists. Practice bulletin no. 145. Antepartum fetal surveillance. https://www.acog.org/Clinical-Guidance -and-Publications/Practice-Bulletins/Committee-on-Practice-Bulletins-Obstetrics/ Antepartum-Fetal-Surveillance. Published July 2014. Reaffirmed 2019.

TRIAL OF LABOR AFTER CESAREAN DELIVERY

Indication
ACOG supports offering women without contraindications a trial of labor after one prior cesarean delivery. Contraindications for trial of labor after cesarean (TOLAC) include the following:[1]

- Prior classical uterine incision
- Prior uterine rupture

- Extensive prior uterine incisions
- Placenta previa

The decision to undergo TOLAC should be reached through shared decision-making between the patient and the provider. Informed consent must include the possibility of uterine rupture and failure to achieve a vaginal delivery. In addition, TOLAC should only be undertaken in a medical facility with the ability to provide emergency surgical intervention.

Equipment
- Tocodynamometer; continuous external fetal heart rate monitoring during a TOLAC is recommended

Procedure
- Patients may present in labor with or without spontaneous rupture of membranes and should be managed accordingly.
- Patients should not receive misoprostol as a cervical ripening agent.
- Patients may receive oxytocin and epidural anesthesia, as appropriate.

> **CLINICAL PEARL:** It is always advisable to discuss the possibility of a TOLAC with the attending physician prior to making a decision.

REFERENCE

1. American College of Obstetricians and Gynecologists. Practice bulletin no. 205. Vaginal birth after cesarean delivery. https://www.acog.org/Clinical-Guidance -and-Publications/Practice-Bulletins/Committee-on-Practice-Bulletins-Obstetrics/ Vaginal-Birth-After-Cesarean-Delivery. Published January 24, 2109.

VAGINAL AND PERINEAL REPAIR AFTER DELIVERY

Indication
During vaginal delivery, lacerations of the vagina and perineum can occur. Lacerations are classified as follows:[1]
- First degree: Injury to skin and subcutaneous tissues of the vagina and perineum without muscle involvement
- Second degree: Injury that extends in to fascia and muscle without anal sphincter involvement
- Third degree: Injury that extends through the fascia and muscle and involves the external and/or internal anal sphincter

- Fourth degree: Injury that involves perineal structures, the internal and external anal sphincter, and rectal mucosa

Equipment
- Sterile gloves and drapes
- Solution for irrigation
- Needle holder
- Suture scissors
- Metzenbaum scissors
- Absorbable sutures (e.g., polyglactin or monofilament 2/0 and 3/0)
- Forceps with teeth
- 1% local anesthetic without epinephrine
- 10-mL syringe
- 22-G needle

Procedure (for 1st- and 2nd-degree lacerations)
1. Inject 1% anesthetic into areas where sutures will be placed.
2. Adequately irrigate the laceration(s).
3. Identify the apex of the laceration.
4. Place an anchoring suture about 1 cm above the apex and use a running stitch to close the vaginal mucosa and underlying fascia.
5. The running suture ends at the hymenal ring and tied.
6. Third- and fourth-degree lacerations should be closed by a surgeon.
7. Ensure adequate hemostasis has been achieved.

REFERENCE

1. Leeman L, Speerman M, Rogers R. Repair of obstetric perineal lacerations. *Am Fam Physician.* 2003;68(8):1585–1590. https://www.aafp.org/afp/2003/1015/p1585.html

9

Common OB/GYN Abbreviations and Terms

Commonly used terms and abbreviations you must know.

ACOG: American College of Obstetricians and Gynecologists

AFI: Amniotic fluid index; an ultrasonic measurement of the sum of the deepest pocket of fluid in all four uterine quadrants; normal is 5 to 24 cm

AMA: Advanced maternal age; defined as a pregnant patient 35 years or older

Amnio. Short for *amniocentesis*

Apgar Score. See the following chart; newborns are assessed at 1 and 5 minutes and assessment can be repeated every 5 minutes if newborns are in distress and resuscitative measures are being utilized

	0	1	2	Total
Activity (muscle tone)	Absent, limp	Some flexion	Active	
Pulse	Absent	< 100 bpm	> 100 bpm	
Grimace (reflex irritability)	Flaccid	Some flexion of extremities	Sneeze, cough, cry	
Appearance (color of skin)	Pale, blue	Trunk pink, extremities blue	Pink	
Respiration	Absent	Irregular, slow	Vigorous cry	
				0–3: Severely depressed
				4–6: Moderately depressed
				7–10: Excellent condition

AROM: Artificial rupture of membranes, or amniotomoy; when the amniotic sac is ruptured with a sterile instrument in order to augment labor

Aromatase inhibitor: Inhibits the conversion of androgens to estrogen; used in in vitro fertilization (IVF) protocols, endometriosis, and in estrogen-receptor-positive breast cancer

Asherman's syndrome: A sequelae of uterine surgical instrumentation whereby intrauterine adhesions (also called *synechiae*) cause amenorrhea and infertility

AUB: Abnormal uterine bleeding; uterine bleeding that does not occur at regular intervals and does not last the typical 3 to 5 days

Blighted ovum: Another term for *anembryonic pregnancy*; the gestational sac will be empty

Braxton–Hicks contractions: Mild uterine contractions that can begin around 28 weeks, do not cause any cervical change, and are typically relieved with activity

Breech presentation: When the fetal caput is not in vertex position; can present as a footling breech or with fetal buttocks

BSO: Bilateral salpingo-oopherectomy; asurgical procedure whereby the uterus and the ovaries are removed; if the ovaries are removed in a woman who is still premenopausal, this will result in an abrupt onset of surgical menopause

BTL: Bilateral tubal ligation; this is typically done laparoscopically; the fallopian tubes are not just ligated, however; they can be cut and cauterized

BUS: Bartholin's glands, urethra, Skene's gland; some providers will document the external genital exam with BUS followed by a short description of findings

Cephalic presentation: Head down position of the fetus

Cephalopelvic disproportion: A term used when the fetal head or body seems too large to pass through the maternal pelvis

Chadwick's sign: A bluish discoloration of the cervix, vagina, and vulva due to increased vascularity in pregnancy

Chancre: A painless, nontender ulceration on an indurated base, usually occurring on the vulva; considered the characteristic finding in primary syphilis; in patients with high-risk sexual behaviors, any genital ulcer should prompt syphilis serologic testing

Chancroid: A tender, erythematous papule that progresses to an ulcer; found on the vulva or perineum and usually painful suppurative inguinal lymphadenopathy is present; caused by *Haemophilus ducreyi*, a Gram-negative rod; chancroid is sexually transmitted, reportable, and partners must be treated as well; the Centers for Disease Control and Prevention (CDC) recommends treatment with 1 g of azithromycin or 250 mg of ceftriaxone

Cholestasis of pregnancy: Caused by bile acid accumulation in the liver causing pruritus and sometimes jaundice; the classic presentation is a patient with generalized pruritus but severe pruritus of the palms of the hands and the soles of the feet; labs will show increased alkaline phosphatase, bile acids (deoxycholic acid, cholic acid, and chenodeoxycholic acid), bilirubin, and sometimes alanine aminotransferase (ALT) and aspartate aminotransferase (AST); bile acids >40 nmol/L are associated with poor prognosis

CIN: Cervical intraepithelial neoplasia; a pathologic diagnosis from tissue taken during colposcopy and biopsy

CKC: Cold knife conization of the cervix for high-grade cervical dysplasia

Colpo: Short for *colposcopy*

Complete Ab (abortion): The cervix is dilated and the patient has expelled products of conception (POC)

Congenital adrenal hyperplasia: The patient usually has congenital masculinization of female genitalia or ambiguous genitalia, and almost all females have a 21-hydroxylase deficiency

Corpus luteum: During the luteal phase of the menstrual cycle, the corpus luteum forms and secretes progesterone and some estrogen; in early pregnancy, the corpus luteum will continue to secrete progesterone until the placenta secretes sufficient amounts; if no pregnancy occurs, the corpus luteum will degrade

Corpus luteum cyst: When the corpus luteum grows to greater than 3 cm, it is called a *corpus luteum cyst*; some can grow very large and cause pain and even ovarian torsion, but the vast majority will regress on their own within a few months

Cotyledon: The slightly bulging, villous, divided areas on the maternal surface of the placenta

CRL: Crown–rump length; the measurement of the embryo from the fetal head to the buttocks; used in the first trimester to estimate gestational age and delivery date

Cx Bx: Cervical biopsy

D&C: Dilation and curettage; a surgical procedure in which the cervix is dilated and the lining of the uterus is scraped

D&E: Dilation and evacuation

DCIS: Ductal carcinoma in situ; a preinvasive disease of the breast, commonly found incidentally on a mammogram

DEXA: Dual-energy x-ray absorptiometry; used to measure bone density

DIC: Disseminated intravascular coagulopathy; inappropriate activation of the clotting cascade due to several obstetric conditions such as placentae abruptio, preeclampsia and eclampsia, amniotic fluid embolism, and postpartum hemorrhage; classic lab abnormalities are prolonged prothrombin time (PT) and activated partial thromboplastin time (aPTT), low platelets and fibrinogen, and elevated D-dimer

Di–Di twin gestation: Dichorionic diamniotic, meaning each gestation has its own placenta and amniotic sac

DMPA: Depot medroxyprogesterone acetate; an injectable medication used for contraception; it is a progestin, has no estrogen, and is administered every 12 weeks

EAb: Elective abortion; some people refer to this as a *TAb*, or *therapeutic abortion*; aTAb is typically done for medical reasons, whereas an EAb means the woman decided to end the pregnancy for nonmedical reasons

ECC: Endocervical curettage; performed with colposcopy

Ectopic pregnancy: Implantation of an embryo in any location outside of the uterus

EDC or EDD: Estimated date of confinement or delivery; this is the patient's due date; alimitation of using the last menstrual period (LMP) to estimate the EDD is that is assumes a 28-day cycle; an EDD by a first-trimester ultrasound is used when the LMP is unknown or disputed

Effacement: The shortening and thinning of the cervix that occurs during labor

EFW: Estimated fetal weight; this is an ultrasound measurement

EGA: Estimated gestational age' this can be estimated from the LMP or the ultrasound

EMB: Endometrial biopsy

EMS: Endometrial stripe; this is an ultrasound measurement that reflects the thickness of the endometrium; it can help guide decision-making when a woman presents with irregular bleeding in the absence of pregnancy; a thick endometrium during the early proliferative stage of the menstrual cycle is abnormal, as is a postmenopausal thick and irregular endometrium

Engagement: A term used to describe when the widest part of the presenting fetus has passed through the maternal pelvic inlet

ER negative: Estrogen-receptor negative breast cancer; this tends to grow fast and occurs in premenopausal women

ER positive: Estrogen-receptor positive breast cancer; responsive to anti-estrogen therapy

ERT: Estrogen replacement therapy

Factor V Leiden mutation: An inherited thrombophilia that is associated with an increased risk of deep vein thrombosis

Fetal alcohol syndrome: A fetal dysmorphology resulting from excessive alcohol consumption during pregnancy; classic findings are microphthalmia, microcephalus, a smooth or flat philtrum, short stature, and cardiac abnormalities; can also include cognitive disorders, behavioral disorders, and difficulty sleeping and eating during the newborn period

FHT: Fetal heart tones; FHTs are auscultated with a hand-help Doppler from about 14 weeks' gestation to delivery; normal FHTs in pregnancy run from 120 bpm to 160 bpm, depending on the fetus' sleep and wake cycle

FIGO classification: The International Federation of Gynecology and Obstetrics's staging for vulvar, endometrial, and cervical cancer

Gestation wheel. A small calendar used to determine a due date using the last menstrual period; every clinic will have some of these laying around; if you hear someone refer to *the wheel*, this is what they mean

GC: Gonococcus, gonorrhea

GnRH: Gonadotropin-releasing hormone

Gravida: A pregnat woman; often used with a number to indicate the number of pregnancies the woman has had

Green Journal. The official journal of the ACOG

GTD: Gestational trophoblastic disease; an aberration of fertilization; also called *molar pregnancy*

GTN: Gestational trophoblastic neoplasia; invasive or metastatic GTD

HDN/HDFN: Hemolytic disease of the newborn/hemolytic disease of the fetus and newborn; also known as *erythroblastosis fetalis*; caused by maternal alloimmunization due to Rh (D) incompatibility

Hegar's sign: Softening of the isthmus of the uterus in early pregnancy

HER2: human epidermal growth factor receptor 2. A prognostic indicator in breast cancer. HER2 positive breast cancers tend to grow more rapidly and will require the use of specific chemotherapy, such as trastuzumab (Herceptin).

HG: Hyperemesis gravidarum; a severe form of persistent nausea and vomiting in pregnancy that results in weight loss and electrolyte deficiencies

HRT or HT: Hormone replacement therapy or hormone therapy; usually refers to hormone therapy during menopause

HSG: hHysterosalpingogram; a radiologic test whereby the radiologist injects dye into the uterus via the cervix and takes images of how the dye moves up through the fallopian tubes; it is a way to see whether the tubes have a blockage that could be causing infertility

HSIL: High-grade squamous intraepithelial lesion; a cytological diagnosis resulting from Pap testing

Incomplete Ab (abortion): POC remain in the uterus

Inevitable Ab (abortion): The cervix is dilated and vaginal bleeding is present

IVF: In vitro fertilization

IUD or IUS: Intrauterine device or system; used for contraception; some IUDs are imbedded with progestins; these can also be used for women who have heavy menses

IUFD/FDIU: Intrauterine fetal demise/fetal death in utero

IUGR: iIntrauterine growth restriction; fetal weight less than the10th percentile for gestational age

IUI: Intrauterine insemination

IUP: Intrauterine pregnancy; the pregnancy is in the uterus; this is a sonographic finding

Kallman's syndrome: Causes hypogonadic hypogonadism and anosmia; patients have a diminished response to gonadotropin-releasing hormone (GnRH) stimulation; after puberty, sex steroid replacement is necessary unless the patient has contraindications

LAVH: Laparoscopic assisted vaginal hysterectomy; a hysterectomy that occurs in the operating room, but it is done transvaginally with the aid of a laparoscope

L/C: Long and closed; this describes a cervix that is neither effaced nor dilated

Lecithin/sphingomyelin ratio: A test of amniotic fluid to help determine fetal pulmonary maturity

LEEP: Loop electrosurgical excision procedure; a thin wire loop that cuts like a scalpel to remove a piece of the cervix affected by dysplastic or precancerous cells

Leopold's maneuvers: A systematic way of palpating a gravid uterus, usually after 36 weeks' gestation, to assess the position of the fetus

LGA: Large for gestational age; a fetus is LGA if it is above the 90th percentile for weight

Lie: The relationship of the longitudinal axis of the fetus to the longitudinal axis of the maternal pelvis; the most common lie is longitudinal; other options are oblique and transverse

LMP: Last menstrual period

LNMP: Last normal menstrual period

Lochia: The vaginal discharge that occurs after delivery; usually lasts 4 to 6 weeks and changes from bloody (lochia rubra) to watery with some brown (lochia serosa) to yellowish-white (lochia alba) tinge

LSIL: Low-grade squamous intraepithelial lesion; a cytological diagnosis from Pap testing

LTL: Laparoscopic tubal ligation

Macrosomia (fetal): A newborn weight greater than 4,000 g

Meconium: A newborn's first stool, it is dark greenish to black; if seen during labor and delivery, it could indicate fetal distress and the baby is at risk of inhaling it, called *meconium aspiration syndrome*

Melasma: A spotty hyperpigmentation of the face common in pregnancy and sometimes seen in women who use estrogen-containing contraceptives

Menstrual history: The shorthand for menstrual history is age at menarche × cycle length × number of days of bleeding

MFM: Maternal–fetal medicine; these are the specialists to whom we refer when the pregnant patient has medical complications; often the MFM will perform amniocentesis and chorionic villus sampling as well

MMG: Mammogram

Missed Ab (abortion): Embryonic or fetal demise is present but there is no vaginal bleeding or cervical dilation

Mono–di twin gestation: Monochorionic diamniotic; refers to one placenta but two amniotic sacs

Mono–mono twin gestation: Monochorionic monoamniotic; refres to one amniotic sac and one placenta

Multip: Multiparous or mutlipara; a patient who has delivered more than one baby

NST: Nonstress test; see section on antepartum fetal assessment in Chapter 4, Diagnostic Testing for OB/GYN Conditions

NSVD: Normal spontaneous vaginal delivery; when the patient delivers vaginally without assistance with forceps or vacuum; some providers use this term to also describe a vaginal delivery that was not artificially induced

Nuchal cord: When the umbilical cord is wrapped 360 degrees around the neck of the fetus; this is common and usually benign unless the cord is wrapped tightly around the neck; as soon as the head is delivered, the obstetrician will alleviate the nuchal cord

Oligohydramnios: An amniotic fluid index less than or equal to 5 cm

Pannus: A large, protuberant, adipose abdomen that can hang over the symphysis pubis that is often a site for localized fungal infections; women who have a large pannus and undergo a cesarean delivery or abdominal hysterectomy can develop a secondary bacterial infection due to hygiene challenges

Para: Number of term deliveries; note that a multiple gestation only counts as one delivery

Pessary: A device that is inserted into the vagina to provide support of pelvic organs, such as when uterine prolapse, bladder prolapse (cystocele), and/or rectal prolapse (rectocele) occurs; there are multiple types of pessaries that can be used, depending on the underlying problem

PG: Phosphatidylglycerol; a constituent of surfactant used to help assess fetal pulmonary maturity

PID: Pelvic inflammatory disease; usually caused by gonorrhea or chlamydia

Placental inspection: A normal human placenta measures approximately 22 cm in diameter, is 2 to 2.5 cm thick, and weighs about 1 pound; both the maternal and fetal surfaces of the placenta must be inspected; the maternal surface is usually dark reddish-maroon; the lobules are called *cotyledons*; all cotyledons should be present without any missing parts; the fetal surface is a grayish translucent color but the reddish-maroon villous tissue underlying it should be seen through the fetal surface; the umbilical cord can measure up to 60 cm and the diameter is up to 2.5 cm; Wharton's jelly is the gelatinous substance covering the cord; the cord is inspected for thromboses or knots and the presence of two arteries and one vein

POC: Products of conception; these arethe tissues from a nonviable pregnancy

Polyhydramnios: An amniotic fluid index greater than 24 cm

Position: The relationship of the back of the fetus' head to the maternal pelvis; the most common is left occiput–anterior (LOA); other positions are right or left occiput–posterior and occiput–transverse

Pouch of Douglas: The area between the cervix and rectum posteriorly and the cervix and vagina anteriorly; also called the *cul-de-sac*

PPH: Postpartum hemorrhage; this is a medical emergency

PPROM: Premature prelabor rupture of membranes; when the amniotic sac spontaneously ruptures before 37 weeks' gestation

Primip: Primiparous or primipara; refers to a woman's first delivery

PR negative (also called *PgR negative*): Breast cancer that is not responsive to progesterone and tends to grow faster than other cancers; patients with ER positive but PR negative breast cancer tend to have more aggressive disease that is resistant to treatment with the selective estrogen modulator tamoxifen

PROM: Prelabor rupture of membranes; when the amniotic sac spontaneously ruptures after 37 weeks' gestation but before the onset of contractions

PR positive (also called *PgR positive*): Breast cancer that is responsive to progesterone

PTL: Preterm labor

PUPP(P): Pruritic urticarial papules and plaques of pregnancy; usually occurs in the latter part of the third trimester; lesions are generally located on pre-existing striae and on the extremities; the rash classically spares the periumbilical region; this does not cause harm to the fetus, and antihistamines can be used to treat the pruritus

RBOW: Rupture of bag of water (see ROM)

Recurrent abortion: Three or more miscarriages, usually consecutive; commonly called *recurrent pregnancy loss*

REI: Reproductive endocrinology and infertility; a subspecialty of OB/GYN that addresses issues of reproduction and infertility

ROM: Rupture of membranes; this refers to the rupture of the amniotic sac

SAb: spontaneous abortion or miscarriage

Septic Ab (abortion): An induced termination of pregnancy that results in infection; the patient is at risk for sepsis

SERM: Selective estrogen receptor modulator; a pharmacologic classification of drugs that vary in their agonist and antagonist effects on different tissues; the SERM tamoxifen is used in the prevention of breast cancer in certain high-risk individuals and for the treatment of ER/PR positive breast cancers.

SGA: Small for gestational age

SROM: Spontaneous rupture of membranes.

SUI: Stress urinary incontinence; loss of urine when the patient coughs or sneezes

SVD: Spontaneous vaginal delivery

TAH: Transabdominal hysterectomy

Threatened abortion: At risk for miscarriage; the cervix will be closed

TOL: Trial of labor

TOLAC: Trial of labor after cesarean

TORCH syndrome: Congenital infection in the newborn that stands for — toxoplasmosis; other infections such as coxsackie, syphilis, varicella zoster, HIV, and parvovirus B-19; —rubella; cytomegalovirus; herpes virus

TPAL: A system used to describe obstetrical history; T is for the number of term births, P is for the number of preterm births (<37 weeks), A is for the number of abortions (miscarriages or elective), L is the number of living children

Trimester: A period of 3 months; pregnancy is divided into three trimesters: the first trimester is from the LMP to 12 weeks, 6 days; the second trimester is from 13 weeks to 26 weeks, 6 days; the third trimester is 27 weeks to delivery

Triple-negative breast cancer: Malignant cells that do not have progesterone or estrogen receptors and do not overly express the protein HER2; more common in younger women and tends to be more aggressive than other types of breast cancer

Trisomy 18: Also known as *Edwards syndrome*; a chromosomal condition caused by an error in cell division

Uterine tachysystole: The presence of more than five uterine contractions in 10 minutes; this is usually an average taken over a 30-minute time frame; it is imperative to pay attention to fetal response to uterine contractions as decelerations could be a sign of fetal distress

UTZ or US: Ultrasound; there are two ways to perform a pelvic ultrasound: transabdominally and transvaginally; you always want to order or perform a transvaginal ultrasound during the first trimester of pregnancy and to adequately evaluate the adnexa if the patient is not pregnant; it is also the preferred way to evaluate the endometrial stripe

UUI: Urge urinary incontinence; a sudden urge to urinate, "when I gotta go, I gotta go right now!"

VAD: Vacuum-assisted delivery

VBAC: vaginal birth after cesarean delivery

VIN: Vulvar intraepithelial neoplasia

VTX: Vertex position of the fetus; ead down; also called *cephalic*

Index